Health Essentials

Natural Beauty

Sidra Shaukat is a qualified make-up artist from a leading international school of make-up based in London. She has given many talks and demonstrations on this subject. Her dissatisfaction with commercial beauty products led her to write this book. She works as a freelance writer on health and beauty, and lives in London.

GW00702691

The Health Essentials Series

There is a growing number of people who find themselves attracted to holistic or alternative therapies and natural approaches to maintaining optimum health and vitality. The *Health Essentials* series is designed to help the newcomer by presenting high quality introductions to all the main complementary health subjects. Each book presents all the essential information on each therapy, explaining what it is, how it works and what it can do for the reader. Advice is also given, where possible, on how to begin using the therapy at home, together with comprehensive lists of courses and classes available worldwide.

The *Health Essentials* titles are all written by practising experts in their fields. Exceptionally clear and concise, each text is supported by attractive illustrations.

Series Medical Consultant
Dr John Cosh MD, FRCP

In the same series

Acupuncture by Peter Mole
Alexander Technique by Richard Brennan
Aromatherapy by Christine Wildwood
Ayurveda by Scott Gerson
Chi Kung by James MacRitchie
Chinese Medicine by Tom Williams
Colour Therapy by Pauline Wills
Flower Remedies by Christine Wildwood
Herbal Medicine by Vicki Pitman
Kinesiology by Ann Holdway
Massage by Stewart Mitchell
Reflexology by Inge Dougans with Suzanne Ellis
Self-Hypnosis by Elaine Sheehan
Shiatsu by Elaine Liechti
Spiritual Healing by Jack Angelo
Vitamin Guide by Hasnain Walji

Health Essentials

NATURAL BEAUTY

The Natural Approach to Skin and Body Care

Sidra Shaukat

ELEMENT

Shaftesbury, Dorset ● Rockport, Massachusetts
Brisbane, Queensland

© Sidra Shaukat 1992

Originally published as *Health Essentials: Skin and Body Care*
by Element Books Limited in 1992

First published in Great Britain in 1996 by
Element Books Limited
Shaftesbury, Dorset SP7 8BP

Published in the USA in 1996 by
Element Books, Inc
PO Box 830, Rockport, MA 01966

Published in Australia in 1996 by
Element Books Limited
for Jacaranda Wiley Limited
33 Park Road, Milton, Brisbane 4064

Cover illustration courtesy © of Telegraph Colour Library
Cover design by Max Fairbrother
Typeset by WestKey Limited, Falmouth, Cornwall
Printed and bound in Great Britain by
Biddles Ltd., Guildford and Kings Lynn

British Library Cataloguing in Publication
data available

Library of Congress Cataloging in Publication Data

ISBN 1 - 85230 - 851 - 6

Note from the Publisher

Any information given in any book in the *Health Essentials* series is not intended to
be taken as a replacement for medical advice. Any person with a condition requiring
medical attention should consult a qualified medical practitioner or suitable
therapist.

Contents

Acknowledgements

I am most grateful to Christine Wildwood for allowing me to use the basic moisturizer formula and some illustrations from her book *Aromatherapy*, also in this *Health Essentials* Series.

I would also like to thank my friends who have given me a few of their favourite treatments, for inclusion in this book.

Last, but not least, I would like to thank my family for their support and encouragement.

Introduction

Before I developed an holistic approach to skin and body care, I would describe myself as a 'beauty freak'. I spent hundreds of pounds trying out each and every product that came on the market. Of course, I could blame my obsession on my training for a diploma in fashion photographic make-up, which required me to assemble a make-up box. Naturally, only the most expensive and prestigious products could help in this very competitive field.

The turning point came when I was preparing to go on holiday to my birthplace in Pakistan. I like to travel light, and when I came to pack my beauty bag, I realized that I needed only the absolute essentials – everything else was unnecessary. I found that all the other products were a waste of money, resources (the Earth's) and space. The extravagant packaging, which accounts for about 10 per cent of the price, makes every purchase mean that you are literally throwing away money, and the products themselves are made of complex, highly processed chemicals, which can cause allergies and adverse reactions. I threw away the products, determined to find natural substitutes.

While I was in Pakistan, I noticed that women in general, including my family and friends, were all beautiful. They had perfect skin and teeth, shiny hair and sparkling eyes, but they did not use expensive moisturizers, treatments and conditioners, which are not even available there, and they did not ever visit the beauty salon! They did not have access to sophisticated beauty products, and yet they were still beautiful.

I came to the conclusion that being beautiful does not require the most expensive, sophisticated products. In fact, in most cases, the simplest products and methods are the most effective.

After my holiday, I grew increasingly to dislike the complex beauty products that are offered for sale. I was determined to find natural products that would be just as effective as the more costly, synthetic products. This is when I began to look into the ancient, time-honoured remedies used by my parents and grandparents. I am fortunate to come from a cultured family from Lahore, Pakistan. This bustling, lively city, with its rich heritage, has combined many different cultures, which has given a wealth of tried and tested beauty remedies.

My mother used to massage olive or coconut oil into my hair and scalp when I was a child, and I think this has resulted in my head of thick, healthy hair. I have often used Dhandasa, a natural tooth brightener, which originates from the bark of a tree; this is chewed and then rinsed away. The traditional Pakistani turmeric and yoghurt skin mask is still used on the bride before her wedding to cleanse her skin, and it is highly effective if used weekly. Natural methods of massage to relieve everyday tension and stress have been passed on through our family. Add to this the importance of a healthy, natural, freshly prepared diet, and it seems that grandma certainly knew best! I also knew of the beneficial properties of fruits, vegetables, herbs and many basic household products. I now wanted to put these ideas into practice and see whether the old remedies really worked. While I was experimenting, I also invented some beauty treatments of my own.

I was so impressed with the effectiveness of these natural, inexpensive beauty treatments that I decided to share my secrets with everyone by writing this book. The list of Absolute Essentials on page 5 includes ingredients that are present in every household. Pampering yourself by using the simple, natural treatments in this book will certainly help you to improve your appearance and your self-esteem. Carrying out the treatments in this book will, in addition, save time, money, space, waste, inconvenience and trips to the shops, but most of all, you will use products that are natural and that are unlikely to cause adverse reactions. Have fun trying out these effective treatments!

1

Skin and Body Care: The Natural Approach

My emphasis in this book is on the natural, holistic way to beauty. Holistic skin and body care takes into account the whole person, the mind-body-spirit concept, on the basis that each aspect is interrelated. Conventional beauty treatments tend to concentrate on only one particular 'problem' – a 'wrinkle', for example – a technique that according to the Greek philosopher Plato, is incorrect: 'The cure of the part should not be attempted without the treatment of the whole'.

This book aims to follow Plato's principle by looking at natural treatments for skin and body care, as well as considering the important aspects of the mind and spirit. It is only by looking at all these aspects that one can achieve true well-being and radiate that special glow that is the sign of real health and vitality.

Many books on skin and body care tend to focus on isolated treatments that are complicated, expensive and time-consuming, that use products that have been tested on animals, and contain animal by-products (slaughterhouse 'excess') and that can cause allergies and skin sensitivity. Even the few books that are available on 'natural beauty' use ingredients that are expensive and difficult to obtain, as well as using complex procedures to make them up.

The treatments in this book, however, use only the simplest ingredients, most of which will already be present in your home – fruit, salt, sugar, for example – so you are sure to reduce your beauty expenditure and avoid inconvenience. It goes without saying that these products are totally cruelty-free, natural and, for the most part, unprocessed.

3

The treatments described are useful for absolutely everyone, regardless of age, sex, race, class or culture. Men, who are becoming increasingly aware of the benefits of good grooming, will certainly find some of the treatments and principles very useful, especially when you consider that most of the grooming and skin care ranges produced for men are actually exactly the same as women's ranges, the only difference being the packaging.

This book is also user friendly. It is simple to understand and to follow: the treatments and techniques are easy to use and the instructions are clear and concise. Even children will have fun making some of the treatments, such as the fruity face masks. Products are made fresh to maximize their effectiveness because the enzymes in fruits such as pineapple and lemon are most efficacious if they are used immediately. In addition, because the treatments are made instantly and 'to order' and you make only as much as you require, there are no problems with waste or storage.

Holistic skin and body care treatments can replace the majority of commercial cosmetics by performing as well as, or better than, shop-bought products. Remember that, because these treatments are natural, they work in harmony with your body, thus minimizing and even eliminating adverse body reactions. You can, nevertheless, hang on to some of your old favourite commercial products if you want to, merely replacing some of them with these natural treatments. It's really up to you.

Some of the treatments are centuries old, and they have not, therefore, required testing on animals. Even some companies that claim they are against animal testing, do not always use completely cruelty-free ingredients. As you will be using essentially organic ingredients that are in their natural state, however, you can rest assured that no animals have suffered for your benefit.

Vegetarians can use these treatments in the full confidence that, unlike commercial cosmetics, they do not contain animal by-products or derivatives. Vegans can use the majority of the treatments, except for those containing eggs. As all the ingredients are clearly stated, vegan readers can easily pick out the unsuitable treatments.

Religions such as Islam, Judaism, Hinduism impose dietary restrictions that apply also to cosmetic products. As most commercial products do not list their ingredients, followers of these religions often have no means of telling if prohibited animal by-products are included. Holistic skin and body care preparations state clearly all ingredients included, so the majority of treatments can be used with complete confidence by members of these religions.

Before we go any further, let us take a look at the type of ingredients you will be using when you work from this book.

THE ABSOLUTE ESSENTIALS

If you want to follow the holistic approach to skin and body care, you will need the following items, many of which will already be present in your home:

Baby oil	Petroleum jelly
Baby powder	Potatoes
Bicarbonate of soda	Salt
Cucumber	Strawberries
Eggs	Sugar
Honey	Teabags
Lemon	Vegetable or sunflower oil
Milk	Water
Oatmeal	Wholemeal flour
Olive oil	Yoghurt

NATURAL INGREDIENTS USED IN HOLISTIC SKIN AND BODY CARE

Almond   Face scrubs and masks made from almonds can eliminate blemishes, blackheads and enlarged pores. Almond balms can moisturize sun-parched and flaky skin.

Apple   One of the oldest beauty aids, apples can be used as the basis of facials, handcreams, hair rinses, tonics and masks. Many germs are unable to survive in apple juice.

Apricot   Vitamin A, in which apricots are rich, is useful in facials, masks and body oils. The oil helps to erase stretch marks and wrinkles.

Avocado   Vitamins A and B, protein and natural oil, and lecithin (a protein that is good for dry and damaged hair) are all found in avocados, which are ideal for nourishing creams and masks.

Banana   Rich in Vitamin A and potassium (germs cannot survive in its presence), bananas are good for cleansing masks and hair treatments.

Bran   When it is used as a facial scrub, the minute and slightly abrasive particles of bran will penetrate deep into pores and remove specks of dirt, grease and dead skin cells.

Carrot   Because they contain vitamin A, carrots are vital for healthy skin. Taken in moderation, carrot juice is good for the complexion, curing and preventing spots, as well as being good for the eyes and hair.

Cucumber   This is used in facial masks to minimize enlarged pores and oiliness and can be used to soothe and heal sunburn.

Egg   Egg whites are astringent and gently stretch the skin, making them a useful addition to masks and creams. Egg yolks are rich in protein, which makes them invaluable in moisturizers for dry, flaky skin. Whole eggs can be used to feed and enrich the hair follicles, giving hair body and shine.

Honey   Honey has been a vital ingredient of beauty preparations since ancient times. Contains high levels of vitamins, minerals and potassium (bacteria cannot survive in its presence), and it soothes, softens and nourishes, making it useful in masks, face creams and hand and body lotions.

Lavender   The antiseptic present in lavender makes it an effective mouthwash. It is also a fragrant and beautifying all-purpose bath ingredient.

Lemon   The acid balance of the skin is disturbed by daily washing, and lemon juice can restore that balance. Pure lemon juice has a drying action, which makes it excellent for oily skins, although people with dry skins should use it only sparingly. Lemon hair rinses are useful for fair-haired people.

Milk   Milk, which is high in protein, calcium and vitamins, is absorbed quickly by the skin, leaving it soft. It is a useful ingredient in cleansing milks, face packs and scrubs and can be added 'neat' to baths.

Oatflakes   The fine and gentle flakes of oat are very effective in removing dirt and grime when they are used in facial masks and scrubs, which leave the skin soft and clean.

Olive Oil   Because it absorbs ultraviolet rays, olive oil is effective as a screening sun-tan lotion. It can also be used to treat damaged hair, dry, flaky skin and weak nails.

Potatoes   A versatile beauty aid, potatoes can be used as a facial cleanser for normal to dry skins. Because they are gentle, they can be applied to swollen eyelids and to sunburnt skin.

Salt   A powerful cleanser, salt is most useful in dentifrices and mouthwashes. Sea salt is a tonic in the bath as well as being a good exfoliator.

Strawberry   An ideal ingredient of face masks, strawberries also have a high pectin content, which makes them very good tooth whiteners if they are eaten raw.

Yoghurt   The acid in yoghurt kills off harmful bacteria on the skin, making it very useful for blemish-prone skin. Yoghurt is used in face masks, scrubs and cleansers. It is also excellent as a hair conditioner or for treating a dry and scaly scalp.

THE COST OF BEAUTY

You have only to think about the cost of beauty for a few minutes to realize why the treatments in this book make sense on every front, including cost.

Each year £32 billion are spent on the diet industry and £28 billion on the cosmetic industry. Of this amount, £4 billion are spent just on make-up, of which £100 million are spent on lipstick alone! An average woman in Britain spends £80 a year on make-up, and the figures are much higher in Continental Europe and the United States.

Some writers have argued that women have to spend so much on 'beauty' because society expects them to conform to an ideal of 'feminine beauty'. It has been suggested that equal opportunities at work have given women so much additional power that the only way in which men can keep them 'in their place' is by persuading them (largely through advertising) that society expects them to conform to an unrealistic 'feminine ideal'.

The treatments in this book are designed to make you, the reader, feel good about yourselves. They do not mean that you have to be a 'slave' to 'beauty'. The emphasis, rather, is on increasing your overall well-being and improving your confidence so that you can project the best image possible, all for a minimal cost and little waste and with the additional benefit of being in harmony with nature.

THE PSYCHOLOGY OF BEAUTY PURCHASING

Next time you are at the cosmetics counter of a large department store or chemist, ask yourself why you have bought a particular product. It is only by assessing your reasons for each purchase that you will be able to eliminate unnecessary and wasteful expenditure. You may have persuaded yourself to buy something for one of the following reasons: 'If I buy the most expensive product, it will be the most effective.' 'I care about my appearance, so I like to spend a lot on it.' 'That woman looks great because she spends so much money on herself.' 'The most expensive items are a status symbol.' 'I loved the pretty box.' 'The model in the advertisement looks so good because she uses those products. If I used those, I could look good too.' 'It's a new product. It's revolutionary. It's hi-tech.' 'All my friends have one, so I should too.' 'I work hard so I deserve to spend a little on luxuries.' 'I've just got to have that particular shade of lipstick.' 'I need to have that purifying mask, as well as the exfoliating one, the moisturizer, the toner and the cleanser, too!'

Cosmetics manufacturers have studied the psychology of women making beauty purchases, and the justification for spending money on expensive products has been researched. The manufacturers sometimes create a need that does not exist, or they will make an existing product more specific – for example, do you really need four types of mask as suggested above?

Your reasons for buying cosmetics may be fickle. You may think that a product looks good on your dressing-table or you may be curious about a new product or a new colour, a two-in-one product or a 'new' formulation. You may want to 'keep up with the Jones', by showing off your latest beauty cream or you may want to have something distinctive in your handbag to show off to friends.

While I am not suggesting that you should never purchase another beauty preparation again, I am asking you to stop for a moment and consider why you should buy the product. There are, of course, some new products that signify genuine advances – the new foundation/powder two-in-one compacts, for example, which are effective, save money and are easy to carry. But what about the rest?

The latest anti-wrinkle creams, for example, should be avoided. Countless doctors and dermatologists have stated that they simply do not work. Most wrinkles are caused by exposure to the sun, and if the anti-wrinkle cream contains UVA/UVB filters to screen out harmful sun rays, then these sun filters alone will make it effective. As we shall see later (chapter 2), skin creams can penetrate only the superficial layers of the skin – they have a 'plumping' effect on the skin, giving it more surface moisture – so any products that claim to alter skin structure radically are simply raising false hopes. Some creams contain highly complex and unusual ingredients. Bovine placenta, for example, can cause allergies and adverse reactions in some people. The natural treatments in this book will do the job just as well, if not better, without causing any unforeseen side-effects or unfortunate reactions.

You may be swayed by the sales talk at cosmetic counters and purchase far more than you need, pay by credit card and have a huge bill to pay next month. To avoid falling into this trap, write a list of all your needs before you go shopping. That's right, your *needs*. Stick rigidly to this list while you are shopping. Learn to say no to those intimidating saleswomen at the cosmetic counters and avoid those costly impulse purchases. Don't think you are making a fool of yourself – after all, you may never see her again! You will find that you will cut down on unnecessary shopping trips and avoid expensive impulse purchases. You will save time, reduce waste and excess, have less wasteful packaging to get rid of and, last but not least, you will save a fair amount of money, too!

TREATMENTS FOR ALL THE FAMILY

Best of all, try to introduce the treatments in this book into your and your family's daily routine. Remember that this book is for all the members of your family. If you do the shopping for them, you can influence them to try the natural treatments in this book instead of their usual products. Try this for a week and you will soon have some enthusiastic converts to the holistic approach to skin and body care.

The trick is not to force these treatments on to the other members of the family but to try subtle persuasion. For example, if your children see you making the fresh fruit face mask (see pages 31-32), no doubt they will want some of this 'magic potion' too!

Leave this book lying around in the living-room for men, teenagers and kids to read at their leisure. At the weekend, try to have a family health day, when you can indulge in your favourite natural treatments from this book. Here are just some of the specific treatments that will be useful for the rest of the family:

Babies   Try gentle massage (see page 77) on the feet and all over the body to relax the baby. Bathe baby in milk and rinse afterwards to keep the skin soft and smooth.

Young Children   They will love having their head and scalp massaged with soothing olive or coconut oil (see page 36). This ensures that their hair will grow thick and healthy as they approach adulthood. Try to persuade them to rinse their mouths with warm salted water after they eat something sweet (see page 52).

Teenagers   Try the deep-cleansing fruit masks, such as pineapple or lemon, in the Weekly Treats for Skin section (pages 31-32). The yoghurt masks, too, are good to help clear up oily skin. The steaming facials once a week will also help to clear up a congested and blocked complexion.

Men   The face masks in the Weekly Treats for Skin section (pages 31-34) will be beneficial. If men apply fresh milk as an aftershave and rinse thoroughly afterwards, they will find that their skin does not sting but will feel soft and smooth. They should also try the treatments for the hair and try scalp massage to control thinning hair (see page 36).

COSMETICS – ENVIRONMENTALLY FRIENDLY?

The media have given considerable coverage to the environment. 'Green issues' and 'environmentally friendly' have become the buzzwords of the 1990s, and there is much discussion about whether paper is recycled or household products contain chemicals that are harmful to the environment. It is, therefore, somewhat surprising that this 'green' trend has not yet filtered through to the major multinational cosmetic companies.

This multi-million pound industry is a large consumer of the world's resources, and yet very few people question its wastefulness. Cosmetic companies spend enormous amounts of money and resources to ensure that their products have the right image. Think of the glossy brochures printed on expensive paper, the elaborate printing of packaging, the expensively produced bottles and jars, not to mention the costly and wasteful resources used to produce the actual contents, just to satisfy you, the sophisticated western consumer.

To illustrate just how wasteful of time, money, space and resources and how environmentally 'unfriendly' the beauty industry is, picture yourself in the following scenario. You run out of your favourite beauty products. Just think how unfulfilled (as a true beauty junkie) your life is without them, so in a panic you drive to the chemist to get them. You use petrol to get there, wasting money and more importantly, adding toxic chemicals, including lead, to the pollution in the air. In addition, you waste time travelling to the chemist, spending time there and returning home. Your purchases will be put in a paper bag or, more wasteful still, a plastic carry bag, and the throw-away receipt will have used paper and ink. You get back home, throw away the paper bag or the carrier bag and discard the cardboard boxes that housed the products (which have taken trees to make and used resources during the printing process). As the packaging costs over 10 per cent of the price, you will have thrown away money and squandered the Earth's resources!

Next come the jars and bottles containing the product. Some containers are 'extras', which can be thrown away immediately; otherwise the container is thrown away when the product is finished. These containers are made by expensive processes that use up energy and chemical resources.

Now consider the actual contents. These may even be cheaper to produce than the expensive, throw-away bottle that contains them! The formulation of the contents would have been arrived at by costly and time-consuming research, which would have wasted the initial raw materials. Then the product would have been manufactured by complex chemical processes, which use up energy, chemicals and scarce resources. Each stage of manufacture would involve several different complex industrial processes before the final product is complete.

The contents may have been tested extensively on animals, which could have resulted in their suffering and death. Even companies that claim they are against animal testing cannot guarantee that they do not use animals in their research. However, the question of animal testing is another issue. Here we will concentrate on the wasting of resources.

Animal tissue and/or proteins may be used, which may be

slaughter-house by-products or they may require further processing, which again wastes resources. Even those companies that insist that all their products are natural, use up valuable resources in the manufacture and packaging.

The alternative to all this is the holistic approach. By using treatments in this book, you will reduce the unnecessary waste of the world's resources. The treatments use only the simplest ingredients, many of which will already be present in your home, and so you are sure to reduce your beauty expenditure and avoid inconvenience. They take the minimum of time to prepare, cut down waste, cost next to nothing, are completely natural, do not contain any animal tissues and are cruelty-free! Now that's what I call environmentally friendly.

2

Your Step by Step Beauty Guide

UNDERSTANDING YOUR SKIN

A beautiful, smooth, soft skin is the ultimate beauty asset, but the skin is also an essential, multi-purpose organ, the largest in the body, in fact, covering around 2.4 sq yards (2 sq m) and weighing between 5½ and 7¾ lb (2.5–3.5 kg).

Your skin protects the vital organs and muscles in your body as well as the delicate sensory organs in the head, such as the eyes. It regulates your body's temperature, increasing sweating if you get too hot and erecting the hair follicles or causing 'goose pimples' if you get too cold. Your skin also disposes of waste matter by means of the sweat glands, thus helping to keep your internal system clean.

The top protective layer, the epidermis, is constantly wearing away and being renewed, as dead skin cells flake off the surface and are replaced by new cells. Your skin renews itself completely every three or four weeks, but this process slows down as you get older. This continuous process ensures that the new layer is tough and resilient. The epidermis is thinnest on the eyelids (hence the need for extra care in this area) and thickest on the soles of the feet and palms of the hands. The outermost layer (the stratum corneum or horny layer) consists of flakes of skin cells, which are overlapped to give a smooth, reflective look to the skin. Exfoliators speed up the renewal of this outermost layer, which is why your skin feels so soft and smooth after exfoliation.

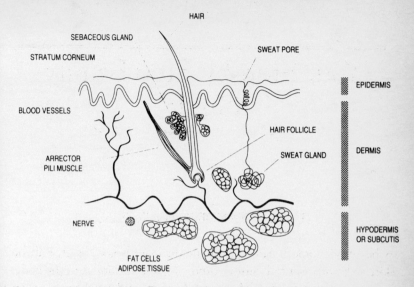

Fig. 1. A cross-section of skin.

Your skin is rather like a waterproof jacket, which protects you from the outside world and prevents dehydration from the inside. Sebum, the body's natural moisturizer, is secreted from the sebaceous glands, and together with moisture released from the epidermal cells, it forms a slightly acidic (around pH 5) layer on the skin to protect it from germs and bacteria. Harsh soaps, which are usually alkaline, astringents and cleansers can attack this protective layer, leaving the skin exposed to infection and more 'sensitive'.

Melanocytes are also present in the skin. These produce melanin, a brownish-black pigment which is responsible for skin colour. Melanin absorbs ultraviolet rays and so acts as a natural sunscreen. The more that skin is exposed to sunlight, the more widespread is the distribution of melanin, so that less ultraviolet light is absorbed by the lower layers of the skin. This is why it is essential to use products containing a sunscreen when out in sunlight.

Below the epidermis is the dermis, which contains the vital fibrous tissues, collagen and elastin, which keep the skin looking young. These fibres act in much the same way as elastic, allowing the skin to move while retaining its shape. When these fibres harden, the skin's

15

elasticity is reduced, giving the characteristic appearance of older skin. The dermis contains blood vessels that supply oxygen to the skin cells and lymph nodes that eliminate waste. Also present are the temperature regulators, sweat glands and ducts, which produce sweat to cool down the body, as well as hair follicles with their sebaceous glands and arrectores pilorum muscles, which make the hairs stand on end to help insulate the body when it is exposed to cold.

Also present in the dermis are nerve endings, which react to changes in the environment and trigger the appropriate responses in the brain. Temperature and touch are detected by the nerve endings – for example, if you pick up something extremely hot, you put it down immediately.

The deepest layer of the skin is the hypodermis or subcutaneous layer, which contains connective tissue and fat cells to protect the body and keep it warm. This fatty layer, or adipose tissue as it is called, varies in thickness throughout the body; it is thinnest on the nose and thickest on the buttocks. Distribution also varies between males and females, with women generally having broader hips and thighs than men.

The hypodermis acts as an energy reserve, which is depleted during starvation, illness, crash diets or prolonged strenuous exercise. It also protects the dermis from the muscles and organs in the body, allowing free movement.

ANALYSING YOUR SKIN TYPE

You may be baffled by the number of skin types that are categorized by the cosmetics industry – normal, dry, sensitive, oily and combination. Which one are you? Skin type has a lot to do with the following factors, some of which are beyond your control:

Heredity　　Along with the colour of your eyes and your hair, you will have inherited your skin type and condition from your parents. So, if your mother was blessed with beautiful skin, the chances are you will be too!

Climate   People who live in hot, dry climates need oily skin with extra sebum (the skin's natural oil) to lubricate and protect it, which is why Afro-Caribbean skin is oilier than European skin. Cool, moist climates result in fine, translucent skin, which is typified by the 'English rose' complexion. However, this has a tendency to become dry.

Age   Your skin will generally be oilier in your youth and will get drier as you age, as sebum output and the skin's natural moisture content decrease.

Other Factors   Environmental factors, such as central heating, air conditioning and pollutants, bodily changes, such as periods, pregnancy, hormonal changes, the menopause and the contraceptive pill, as well as stress, emotional factors and diet can all have an effect on your skin type.

Your skin type may change from oily to sensitive, or from normal to combination. You should keep an eye on your skin type, especially if you begin to develop adverse reactions or become sensitive to a particular product or ingredient.
  Now let us see how you can further analyse your skin type.

Normal Skin   is 'perfect skin'. It is soft, smooth and finely textured, does not flake, become dry or oily or develop spots. Babies and children usually have normal skin, but it needs attention, care, a good diet and the right beauty treatments to keep it that way.

Dry Skin   is close textured and fine, but it can feel tight, flake and is predisposed to developing facial lines. It should not be subjected to extreme weather conditions of hot and cold or to wind. Moisturizers to replace the lack of the natural skin lubricant, sebum, are essential for this skin type.

Sensitive Skin   is fine and translucent, but it can develop lines and small surface veins. It can suffer redness and irritation when exposed to allergens in the air and to products such as perfume, lanolin, pollen or other pollutants. Keep it away from extreme weather and complex cosmetic products.

Oily Skin has a characteristic shiny look and is prone to develop spots. The increased sebum production is generated by the male hormone, testosterone, which is present also in small quantities in women. The skin is thicker and can have enlarged pores, with a tendency towards blackheads and blemishes. Avoid the temptation to use harsh cleansers, which can overstrip the natural oils and hence overstimulate oil production. Gentle cleansing is best to maintain the skin's balance.

Combination Skin is most common between the ages of twenty and forty. The chin, nose and forehead, the T-zone of the face, contain more sebaceous glands and so are oilier than the rest of the face. The skin around the eyes, cheeks and neck will be dry. Do not be tempted to use products made for oily skin on areas other than the T-zone.

Look at the Skin Analysis Chart on page 20 to check which skin type you are. Remember that skin type is not static and your skin will generally become drier with time. If you suffered from spot-prone skin as a teenager, do not dismiss yourself as having oily skin, even though you may be well into your twenties or thirties. Most of all, be honest if you are to treat your skin correctly because products are specifically designed for the skin type stated. Examine your skin in good light, without any make-up, and preferably in a magnifying mirror. Circle the points that best match your skin. For example, if the most circles are in the combination skin column, your overall skin type is combination and you should use products made for combination skins.

TREATING YOUR SKIN TYPE

Now that you have analysed your skin type, you will need to carry out the correct treatments to look after it. You may have favourite products that you have been using for years, which you feel do a great job. In that case, by all means stick with them. If, on the other hand, you wish to try new, natural, cruelty-free products, there are highly effective products that you can make yourself, and some of these are given at the end of this chapter.

Normal Skin

You are lucky to have normal skin, so keep it that way by treating it with tender, loving care. Never take it for granted. Use gentle cleansers, toners and moisturizers daily and use a face mask once a week.

Dry Skin

Keep this fragile skin away from extremes of temperature and from wind. Avoid soap and instead use gentle cleansers, alcohol-free toners and day moisturizers. Always use a night cream. Use a moisturizing face mask once a week.

Sensitive Skin

Sensitive skin should be kept away from all possible allergens in the air and in cosmetic products. Use cleansers, toners and moisturizers that are alcohol-free, fragrance-free and, preferably, lanolin-free. Do not use complex, anti-wrinkle creams containing synthetic, over-processed chemicals because these can trigger adverse reactions, and you should, preferably, avoid face masks and facial scrubs.

Oily Skin

Oily skin can become 'problem skin', so do not resort to using harsh products, which can make the problem worse. Use either a mild, pH-balanced soap or a cleanser, toner and oil-free moisturizer. Apply a facial scrub once or twice a week and a deep-cleansing face mask once a week. Some oily skins can benefit from a weekly steaming session.

Combination Skin

Do not fall into the trap of treating this skin as if it were oily skin. Use gentle cleansers and toners and oil-free moisturizers, paying particular attention to the drier areas. Give yourself a facial scrub once a week on the T-zone of the nose, forehead and chin and a gentle face mask once or twice a week.

Skin Analysis Chart

Do you have?	Normal	Dry	Oily	Sensitive	Combination
Large pores			✔		✔
Fine texture	✔	✔		✔	
Shiny nose			✔		✔
Shiny T-zone			✔		✔
Shiny face			✔		
Tightness		✔		✔	
Flaky skin		✔		✔	
Redness				✔	
Acne			✔		
Spots			✔		✔
Blackheads			✔		✔
Thread veins		✔			
Facial lines		✔			
Wrinkles		✔			
Thin skin		✔		✔	
Thick skin			✔		✔
Tanned skin			✔		✔

Whatever your skin type, you should use an eye gel, applied gently on the eye area, a lip balm and preferably a sunscreen when you are going out of doors for any length of time.

A BASIC DAILY SKIN CARE ROUTINE FOR EVERYONE

A basic routine is essential for keeping your skin healthy, clean and soft. Stick to your routine religiously if you want to see the best results; don't just do it when you feel like it. Perform the routine first thing in the morning and last thing at night. Always be gentle to your skin and avoid dragging or stretching your skin to prevent lines from forming.

If you are starting a daily skin care routine and you want to stick to your favourite commercial products, you should use products of the same make and range, because they are designed to work well together. However, try substituting the commercially produced cosmetics with the natural, simple and economical products you can make yourself from the recipes at the end of this chapter. You will see they work just as well, if not better!

Cleansing

Cleansing is the first part of your routine. Its purpose is to dislodge dirt, sweat and make-up from deep within the skin. Some people think that cleansing is meaningless if they do not splash themselves with water; others find water-cleansing too harsh. The trick is to use gentle products and to stick to those that suit you best. See my recipes (on pages 27-28) for gentle cleansing products you can make yourself.

A wide variety of cleansers is available, ranging from the simplest of soaps to the most expensive cleansing lotions. Soaps can be used by everyone provided that they are pH-balanced and so do not strip the skin of its protective acidic layer. Soap-free gels are also good for everyone, although they may not effectively deep cleanse oily skin.

Cold creams can be too heavy on fine, delicate skin, and they can drag the skin; they can also leave some residue behind. The cold cream recipe given on page 28 is light, and, because it contains almond oil, it is beneficial for all skin types, even dry skins. It goes on smoothly and avoids any pulling or stretching of the skin, which can happen with commercial cold creams.

Cleansing lotions, rather than creams, should be used for dry skins because they can be applied with a lighter touch. Warm up the lotion in the palms of your hands, then massage it gently into the skin. Wipe off gently with a soft facial tissue or cotton wool.

Toning

Toning cools the skin, removes the last traces of cleanser and prepares the skin for moisturizing. Some toners contain alcohol and can be harsh for all skin types. Stick to alcohol- and perfume-free toners, which are suitable for everyone. Apply with a cotton wool pad, preferably two, and use one for each side of the face for maximum hygiene.

Moisturizing

Moisturizing is essential, even for people with oily skins. Moisturizers can be in liquid form or thick cream form, and although thick creams are suitable for dry skin, some kinds can drag the skin and accentuate lines, while liquid moisturizers are useful for everyone. Apply moisturizer lightly to the face with your fingertips, being especially careful around the eye area, (which should only be treated with gels or moisturizers specifically developed for this area).

Protecting Your Skin

Always include an eye gel and lip balm in your daily skin care routine. The skin around the eyes is the thinnest of the whole body, and the lips have very few sebaceous glands. Both these areas, therefore, require extra special gentle care. In addition, because of the damage caused to the ozone layer, you should protect your skin from the potentially carcinogenic ultraviolet rays of the sun by applying a sunscreen whenever you are likely to be exposed to sunlight.

Eye Gel
Be very careful around the delicate skin of the eyes because this area is one of the first to show the signs of ageing such as fine lines and wrinkles. Every morning and evening gently apply an eye gel with your little finger around the bone of the eye socket. You can use a commercially prepared, preferably fragrance- and alcohol-free, product or you could try wheatgerm oil instead.

Lip Balm
To avoid dry lips, always use a lip balm as often as you wish throughout the day but always when you go outdoors and at night. If you use a balm under your lipstick, it will make the lipstick go on smoothly,

prevent the lipstick from staining your lips and make the lipstick last longer.

Petroleum jelly is by far the best lip balm, but you could try making your own, using this simple recipe. Use one part beeswax to one part coconut, almond, jojoba or wheatgerm oil (whichever you prefer). Melt the beeswax over gentle heat and blend in the oil. Allow to cool and apply directly to your lips.

Sunscreen

Olive oil absorbs the burning ultraviolet rays of the sun and is an excellent screening sun lotion. Use it whenever you are sunbathing, but do be careful not to over-do sun exposure. Alternatively, if you prefer to use a commercial product, you should select the correct sun protection factor (SPF), although this can be something of a matter of trial and error. If you are in doubt, choose a higher protection factor rather than a lower one. As a rule, if you have fair or red hair and a fair skin you will require more protection than people with dark hair and darker skins.

If you wear make-up, use a sun-block as a protective base for your skin before you apply your make-up, although many foundation creams and moisturizers now have sunscreens added to them. The sunscreen will not only protect your skin from the harmful and ageing ultraviolet light from the sun but will provide an extra shield against other pollutants in the atmosphere.

Removing Make-Up

Always remove all make-up, especially at night. The above skin care routine should be sufficient to remove most make-up, but some make-up is particularly stubborn, especially waterproof mascara.

The easiest way to remove mascara gently is to dip a cotton wool bud (using one end for each eye) in baby oil, then gently stroke the oil on to your eyelashes to remove every trace of mascara. Use more cotton buds if necessary. In fact, baby oil is perfect to remove all stubborn traces of make-up. Rinse afterwards with toner if you don't want to leave the oil on the skin (it can irritate those with sensitive eyes). If you do not want to use baby oil, sweet almond oil is a good substitute.

At-a-glance Skin Care Chart

Skin Care Routine	Normal	Dry	Oily	Combination	Sensitive
Cleanser	Lotion	Cream	Lotion	Lotion	Lotion
Toner	Mild	Alcohol-free	Deep-cleansing		Alcohol-free
Moisturizer	Lotion	Cream	Oil-free	Lotion	Fragrance-free
Night cream		Essential			
Face mask (pw)	1	1	2	2	1
Steaming (pw)	1	Avoid	1–2	1	1 (if ok)
All skins should use a lip balm, eye gel and body moisturizer daily.					

NOTE: pw = per week

SPECIAL SKIN CARE NEEDS

Everyone's skin requires special care to keep it at its best, and over the years the needs of babies, young children, teenagers and the elderly will change. Men, too, have special skin care needs, and they are only just becoming more interested in looking after their skins.

Babies

No doubt you will have heard the phrase 'as smooth as a baby's bottom'. Well, this is absolutely true, because a baby's skin (especially the bottom) is protected from the outside world, hence the skin is smooth. Babies are also free from the hormonal changes that occur throughout adolescence and adulthood and that affect the skin's condition and appearance.

It is best to use only those products that have been designed especially for babies. Always keep the skin around the nappy area very dry by using baby powder. Bathe frequently using a baby bath cleanser or oil. Avoid using perfumed products because these can cause adverse reactions.

Young Children

Young children still have beautiful skins, but they will not be protected from the outside world to the same extent as babies. Whenever they are in the sun, children should always wear a sun-block or cream with a sunscreen in it. Do not keep the sun-protection for yourself. Make sure that the product contains filters for both UVA and UVB rays to protect the skin against sunburn and premature ageing (see page 23).

As far as other products go, children can continue to use gentle baby formulations for their delicate skins. Young children should never use products designed for adults' skins.

Teenagers

This is probably the most difficult time for the skin, and at this stage it should be treated with the utmost care. At puberty, the hormonal levels of girls and boys are changing as they go through the process of becoming adults. The male hormone, testosterone (which is present in girls, too), is responsible for increasing facial and body hair, and it also thickens skin and increases the production of sebum, making it oilier.

This is a worrying period at best, but if acne or spots start to develop, any emotional problems can be made worse. It is best to seek medical advice as soon as a case of acne occurs, instead of trying to treat it at home by using all the products available on the market and possibly causing permanent acne scars. Your doctor will prescribe oral antibiotics, Retin-A cream (a new treatment, which is effective in some cases) or, for girls, female hormones. The sufferer should stick to medically prescribed treatments.

Only gentle soaps, cleansers and toners should be used, not the harsh, alcohol-based astringents often seen on the market, which strip the skin of the protective acidic layer and the skin's natural oils. An oil-free moisturizer should be used.

Ageing Skin

As skin starts to age, it begins to become dry, to develop wrinkles and lines and to start to sag. Using a light moisturizer both day and night is essential to replace the loss in the skin's natural oils. The facial exercises described in this book will also help to improve muscle tone and thereby the appearance of the skin.

Use moisturizing creams that are not too heavy, and avoid anti-wrinkle creams, which are basically refined moisturizers with chemical additives. Do not use soaps, which are far too drying for ageing skin, and try a moisturizing mask once a week.

Men

Men have facial hair that is continually growing, hence requiring constant shaving. Men with beards are effectively protecting their skin from the outside world, and so, while their foreheads might develop lines, the skin under the beard will be relatively smooth.

The process of shaving essentially strips the skin of its outermost layer, thereby speeding up skin renewal, and this is why men tend to age better than women. If aftershaves are used, they should ideally be moisturizing and not too harsh. Men's skins are oilier and thicker than women's, so they should steam their faces once a week.

MAKING YOUR OWN CLEANSERS, TONERS AND MOISTURIZERS

You can make your own natural cleansers, toners and moisturizers for a fraction of the cost of commercial products, with the minimum of waste and the additional advantage of knowing the exact ingredients.

You can also tailor-make them to your own tastes or requirements. Use them within a month so that they retain their freshness or make them up fresh as and when required. Always store them in a cool, dry place in airtight containers. It's easy, instant and fun too!

Ingredients

You can obtain most of the following ingredients from chemists at minimal prices; alternatively, try herbalists or health food shops. Ingredients are given in small quantities so that you can try them first before making them up in larger quantities if you wish.

The following ingredients form the basis of most cosmetics:

> Almond oil
> Alum (powdered)
> Borax
> Glycerin
> Orange flower water
> Rosewater
> White and yellow beeswax
> (yellow beeswax is unrefined)
> Witch hazel

Cleansers

Lavender Cleansing Cream for Oily Skin
Contains beeswax, almond oil, lavender oil
To make a cleansing cream for oily/problem skin, you will need 2 tablespoons (40 ml) of grated beeswax to 1 tablespoon (20 ml) almond oil. Melt both together over a low heat. Remove and add 1 drop of lavender oil to 1 tablespoon (20 ml) of water (preferably mineral). Whip vigorously until creamy.

Lemon Milk Cleanser for all skin types, especially Oily Skin
Contains buttermilk, lemon
Whisk 1 tablespoon (20 ml) of buttermilk with 1 tablespoon (20 ml)

of lemon juice and apply immediately with cotton wool. Rinse well with tepid water.

Cold Cream for all skin types
Contains borax, white beeswax, almond oil
Dissolve ½ teaspoon (3 ml) of borax in 2 tablespoons (40 ml) of mineral water. Melt 1 tablespoon (20 ml) of white beeswax over low heat, stir in 4 tablespoons (80 ml) of almond oil and add the borax solution. Remove from the heat and allow to cool.

Toners

Rosewater on its own makes an effective toner for all skin types. Add ½ teaspoon (3 ml) of glycerin to 2 tablespoons (40 ml) of rosewater for a gentle toner for dry skins. For a deep cleansing toner for oily skins add 1 tablespoon (20 ml) of witch hazel to 1 tablespoon (20 ml) of rosewater.

Astringent Toning Lotion for Dry Skin
Contains rosewater, orange flower water, witch hazel
Whisk 4 tablespoons (80 ml) of rosewater with 1 tablespoon (20 ml) of orange flower water and 1 tablespoon (20 ml) of witch hazel.

Skin Freshener for Normal Skin
Contains alum, rosewater, witch hazel
Dissolve ½ teaspoon (3 ml) of powdered alum in 1 teaspoon (5 ml) of hot water. Add 2 tablespoons (40 ml) of rosewater and 2 tablespoons (40 ml) of witch hazel.

Moisturizers

This basic moisturizing cream is richer and heavier than commercial creams, but it is very effective and economical. It hardens when put in the fridge (which you should do to stop mould forming), but softens on contact with the skin. Add 1 teaspoon (5 ml) of wheatgerm oil (which is a natural preservative) to increase its shelf-life. You will need:

> 1/6oz (5 g) of yellow beeswax
> 2 tablespoons (40 ml) almond oil
> 2 teaspoons (10 ml) of mineral water or rosewater
> 2 drops of essential oil (rose for dry or ageing skin, lavender for oily, normal or sensitive skin) in weak solution of 1/2 per cent concentration (i.e., 2 drops to 1 tablespoon (20 ml) of base oil)

Melt the beeswax and oil in a heat-proof basin over a pan of simmering water. Heat the distilled water in another basin over a pan of simmering water until it is warm. Add the warm water to the oil and wax, drop by drop, beating with a whisk. When you have mixed 1 teaspoon (5 ml) of the water with the oil and water, remove the pan from heat and add all the remaining water a little at a time. As the mixture sets, stir in the essential oil. Bottle in sterilized glass pots and cover.

If you do not want to make your moisturizer from scratch, try purchasing an unperfumed basic moisturizer such as Cream E45. Slowly add a few drops of your favourite essential oil to the cream and blend thoroughly.

WEEKLY TREATS FOR THE SKIN

The following treats really wake up the skin, removing dead skin cells (exfoliation), opening pores and extracting deeply embedded dirt, as well as boosting circulation – they will bring your skin to life!

People with dry and sensitive skins should use the treatments only once a week or once a fortnight and choose only one treatment each for exfoliating, steaming and masks. If you have an oily or combination skin you can get away with using the treatments twice a week as long as your skin does not have a tendency to be 'sensitive'. Try not to overstimulate your skin and use these highly effective treatments sparingly.

When a treatment states the skin type for which it is most suitable, it wise to adhere to this. For example, a mask for dry skins should not be used by someone with oily skin. If you have combination skin, however, use a treatment for oily skin only on the oily area – i.e., the T-zone of the face, which consists of forehead, nose and chin. Use the treatments for dry skin on the cheeks.

Anyone who has sensitive and fragile skin may want to avoid those treatments that contain acidic ingredients such as lemon and pineapple and possibly yoghurt. Exfoliation should be done gently, and use castor sugar instead of granulated sugar in the facial scrub containing sugar (see below).

Exfoliating

Exfoliation, however it is executed, dislodges dead skin cells and speeds up the rate of cell renewal, and it is essential as you get older because your metabolism will slow down. Exfoliate by briskly brushing your skin with a loofah or massage mitt, which will get skin glowing. Alternatively, you can use finely ground oatmeal, a good gentle exfoliator, which makes an effective scrub before a shower. Simply rub it all over your skin.

Slough off dead skin cells with a mixture of 1 dessertspoon (10 ml) of finely ground almonds in a small carton of yoghurt. Massage over a clean complexion, then rinse away to leave your skin fresh and bright. If your skin is sensitive, use oatmeal instead of almonds.

Facial scrubs will clear and brighten the complexion. Try a peach scrub: mash or liquidize in a food processor a large ripe peach, mix in 1 dessertspoon (10 ml) of oatmeal and rub the mixture all over your face. Rinse with warm water.

An inexpensive facial scrub and good exfoliator can be made by mixing a small amount of sugar (preferably a coarse kind such as granulated sugar) with your favourite cleanser. Massage over your face and wash off thoroughly. This acts in the same way as the expensive gels with exfoliating 'beads' in them, but it is also gentler and much cheaper.

A nutty facial scrub can be made by crushing 4oz (100 g) of blanched almonds to a fine paste. Add an egg and 2 teaspoons (10

ml) of rosewater. Mix well. Use your fingertips to ru
gently into the oily areas of your face. Leave it for 10 minutes
rinsing off well.

Grape juice is an effective natural exfoliator, removing dead skin cells and brightening the skin. Grapeseed oil is also a good, light moisturizer for normal to dry skin. Apples, too, are natural skin exfoliators – just cut a slice and whisk it over your face, using gentle, circular movements.

Steaming

Steam unclogs pores to deep cleanse skin and soften it. Use a deep bowl filled with boiling water. Incline your face towards the steam and cover your head with a towel that will also go around the edges of the bowl to prevent steam escaping. The steam will penetrate and open the pores to bring the dirt to the surface. Tone with a non-alcoholic toner applied with cotton wool to close and tighten pores. Repeat weekly.

Tea acts as a mild tonic and conditioner, and a steaming tea facial will deep cleanse the skin. Pour hand hot tea into a bowl, add a few dashes of lemon rind and some marjoram and mint (dried herbs will do). Now lean your face over the bowl and cover your head with a towel. The heat and toning polyphenols in the tea will draw out impurities.

If you have dry skin, you may want to put some jojoba oil or evening primrose oil in the bowl to soften your skin if you are having a steaming session. Your skin will be able to absorb the oil as the pores open because the oil is in the form of tiny droplets.

Face Masks

Dry Skins

Apricot Oil Mask   Apricot kernel oil helps to maintain healthy skin and surface tissue. Because it is lightweight it soaks in quickly, so it is

31

...skin, and it contains vitamin A, which
... it as a face mask for dry skin.
...cloth or muslin into a mask, making holes for
...outh. Dip the cloth in warmed apricot kernel
...ur face. Leave it in position for 10 minutes, before
...fully. Wipe your skin clean, splash your face with
...for a few minutes before applying make-up.

Avocad...sk   Avocado is an oily fruit, and it makes a great tonic
for dry skins. Mash an avocado with a drop of lemon juice to make a
facial mask that will clarify and soften your skin. It contains lots of
vitamins and minerals, which will, literally, feed your skin.

Avocado Night Mask   If you have dry skin, try an avocado night
mask. Mash or liquidize a ripe avocado into a cream, smooth it on to
your face and relax for 15 minutes. Tissue away most of the cream but
leave a trace on the skin's surface. During the night the remaining
oils will condition and soften the skin.

Banana Mask   For dry 'winter' skin, try a soothing banana facial.
Mash a banana, add a teaspoon of honey to bind and a dash of cream.
If you have oily skin use orange juice and another drop of honey. Very
refreshing!

Egg Mask   Whisk an egg white and mix it with 1 teaspoon (5 ml)
of honey. Apply it to your face with a pastry brush and leave for 10
minutes before washing off with cold water. The egg white gives this
mask its firming effect.

Peaches and Cream Mask   For a peaches and cream complexion
make a reviving face mask by mashing a peach and adding a spoonful
of cream. Rinse off with lukewarm water.

Oily Skins

Clay Mask   Make a clay mask by mixing a whisked egg white with
1 tablespoon (20 ml) of fuller's earth (which is available from chemists). Add a few drops of peppermint oil. Leave to dry and rinse with
lukewarm water.

Lemon Mask　　Lemon juice is a well-known cure for sallow, oily skin, and it is an ideal ingredient in face masks. Lemon juice is good for spot-prone skin because it neutralizes bacteria, and it contains high levels of vitamin C, which helps the skin to heal. Rub a slice of lemon over your face skin and rinse with cold water.

All Skin Types

Exotic Fruit Mask　　Fruits such as pineapple and papaya (or pawpaw) make good face masks because of the enzymes they contain, which help in the healing of wounds and are thus natural aids for the skin. Simply mash up the fruit, put it directly on your skin, leave for 10–15 minutes and rinse well to reveal a softer skin.

Kelp Mask　　All skins benefit from a face mask that deep cleanses and refines without irritating. Take 3 tablespoons (60 ml) of powdered kelp (which is available from many herbalists), mix it with a little almond oil and rosewater (which is available from chemists). Apply to clean skin, leave for 10 minutes, rinse off and moisturize. Use weekly.

Strawberry Mask　　Mashed strawberries make a stimulating face mask. Simply cover your face with the fruit purée for 5–10 minutes, then rinse well with tepid water. Apply a gentle toner if required.

Problem Skins

Turmeric Mask　　Many Asians believe that turmeric (a yellow spice available in powder form from most supermarkets) clears problem skins and promotes a smoother, softer complexion. In fact, in some parts of India, it is applied as a paste on both the bride and groom before the wedding to enhance their beauty!

You can mix 1 teaspoon (5 ml) of turmeric with a few drops of warm water or milk and apply directly to the face. Alternatively, you can mix the turmeric with oatmeal (to exfoliate) and 1 teaspoon (5 ml) of yoghurt (which will act on bacteria, thus preventing spots). If you have dry skin you may wish to add a few drops of almond oil. Leave for 15–20 minutes or until it is dry. Wash off with warm water and a mild soap or cleanser (try some of the recipes given), then use a gentle, non-alcoholic toner (see page 28) with cotton wool to remove all traces of any remaining yellow stain. Use once a week, preferably at night, to enhance the skin's regenerating process, and either before or after a steam session to deep cleanse your skin.

Skin Fresheners

A clean face flannel dipped in hot water placed over your face while you are lying down is an instant relaxer. To freshen or revive a tired face, dip a clean flannel in ice-cold water and place it over your face for 5 minutes. Your face will have a healthy, pink glow, signifying increased blood circulation to the surface of the skin. Your eyes will sparkle, too, and any puffiness will be eliminated.

Use cucumber to make several skin fresheners, which will be useful for normal skins, but especially for oily to combination skins. Purée (or grate if it is easier and quicker) a few slices of peeled cucumber with 2 tablespoons (40 ml) of natural yoghurt. Use this as a face mask for 30 minutes and rinse off with lukewarm water. Incidentally, yoghurt and cucumber dips are popular eaten after a hot curry to cool down! Use the leftovers of the dip to make a refreshing face mask!

Treating Occasional Spots and Blemishes

To treat the odd blemish on all skin types dip a cotton bud in witch hazel and dab it directly on the area. At bedtime, soak a cotton wool ball in calamine lotion and apply it directly to the affected area. For stubborn spots, dot a tiny amount of a face pack such as clay, which dries hard, on the spot before going to bed. Toothpaste will also help to dry up spots. Put it directly on the spots with a brush and leave overnight.

Finally, give your skin an instant boost with a spray of mineral water. Fill a plant spray or a refillable perfume spray bottle for your handbag with bottled water and squirt it over yourself whenever your skin feels dull and sweaty. The spray also sets make-up, making it stay put all day!

BATHTIME

Bathing is an excellent way of relaxing after a hard day, but overusing commercial bath preparations can dry out your skin.

Natural Bath Preparations

Herbal baths are a refreshing alternative and are useful for sufferers from cystitis, who should avoid perfumed bubble baths and oils. Tie a handful of fresh herbs in a piece of muslin and fasten it under the bath taps. Run the hot water first to release the scent from the herbs and then top up with cold water. Try lovage, camomile (you could even use camomile or herbal teabags), mint or rosemary. If fresh herbs are not available, you can use dried herbs instead. A drop of baby, wheatgerm or almond oil in the water will stop your skin from drying out.

Sink into a warm bath scented with essential oils – ylang-ylang, patchouli or rosemary (to clear the head) or lavender, rose or camomile (to relax and soothe), for example. Make sure the water is not too hot, because this will overstimulate the nervous system and inhibit the therapeutic powers of the oils. To make this indulgent soak extra special, put on some soft, soothing music, dim the lights in the bathroom and relax.

Meditate in a warm, relaxing bath by closing your eyes, breathing in deeply and thinking beautiful thoughts – for example, you might like to imagine that you are relaxing on a favourite beach, listening to the sound of waves gently lapping on the shore and the breeze whispering in the palm trees overhead. Add a few drops of essential oil such as lavender, marjoram or juniper to increase the skin-soothing properties of your bath. Lavender has a deeply relaxing effect on body and mind.

The scent of orange is considered a pick-me-up and an antidepressant, so it is an ideal perfume to add to the bath at the end of a long, hard day. Add a drop of essential oil of orange or squeeze a seedless orange into the bathwater to refresh yourself and to aid relaxation.

Body or baby oil can also be used as a bath oil. Maximize the moisturizing potential of the oil by soaking in the bath first before adding a few drops of your chosen oil to the water. This will ensure that the oil veils your skin and seals in some of the water absorbed in the soak.

Cleopatra is said to have bathed in ass's milk to enhance her beauty. Instead of ass's milk, try adding ¼ pint (150 ml) of ordinary milk to the running water, or try 2 tablespoons (40 ml) of dried milk for the same effect. For extra indulgence and to give the bath a tropical feel, add a few drops of coconut essence.

Looking After Your Legs

If you want to have silky smooth legs, exfoliate using a vegetable-based soap on a damp loofah or body brush, sweeping it up over wet skin in massaging movements. This will get rid of dead skin cells and loosen sebum blockages in pores. Legs have comparatively few sebaceous glands and are, therefore, prone to dryness. After a bath, slick on plenty of moisturizer, using upward massage movements. The steam from the bath will help to lock in moisture.

If you suffer from exceptionally flaky winter legs try this pack while you are in the bath. Mash an avocado, a banana and 1 tablespoon (20 ml) of thick cream and smooth it on to your skin. Leave for 10 minutes, then rinse off to reveal beautifully smooth legs.

Swollen ankles will be soothed by a solution of 2 tablespoon (40 ml) of Epsom salts in 1¾ pints (1 litre) of lukewarm water. Bathe your feet and ankles for 10 minutes, then immerse them in cold water to reduce the swelling. Pat dry and massage gently until the aching stops.

Scalp Massage

To release tension in your head, try scalp massage while you are in the bath. Start at the front of your head and press your finger tips firmly against your scalp. Gently move the scalp back and forth five times. Repeat, moving your fingers until you have covered your whole head.

Body Scrubs

For an inexpensive body scrub that will effectively smooth away roughness and soften your skin, try sea salt. First, apply a little vegetable oil, such as almond or olive oil, to dampen your skin. Then give yourself a good rub with handfuls of sea salt, concentrating on any dry patches, such as your knees or elbows. Rinse off with a forceful shower of warm water followed by a cold shower to complete the toning treatment.

A bath containing a liberal sprinkling of sea salt is good for easing muscular aches and for curing minor skin problems.

Face packs need not be used only on your face. Try them on other areas of your body such as your shoulders to unclog pores and slough off dead skin.

Clean greasy patches on shoulders and back with a soap-filled backbrush or loofah. If your back is badly blemished, use a deep-cleansing pack made from some fuller's earth mixed with a little water and lemon juice. Leave to dry and rinse off thoroughly with lukewarm water.

Facial scrubs and sponges to exfoliate the face can also be used on neglected areas such as rough knees and elbows. Massage thoroughly, then rinse. Apply a moisturizer or some handcream. (Handcream can be more economical than body lotion and just as effective.)

To treat badly neglected elbows, scrub them with a pumice stone or a bristle brush, then bleach them with lemon juice. Alternatively, try resting your elbows in two squeezed-out halves of a lemon. Smooth the skin afterwards by rubbing in plenty of moisturizer or your favourite oil.

3

Beauty Highlights:
Treatments for Specific Areas

HAIR

Your hair reflects your state of health and your emotional well-being. Hair grows at a rate of ½ inch (12 mm) a month and has a lifespan of from three to six years. Each strand originates in a bulb-like follicle beneath the surface of the skin and is made up of three layers: the cuticle (a protective outer layer), the medulla (an inner hollow core) and the cortex, strengthened by the protein keratin, which lies between. Hair renews itself and therefore responds well to the treatments outlined here.

Spend as much time as you can exercising outdoors, because the combined effects of exercise, such as walking, and fresh air can work wonders by increasing oxygen supply to the scalp and thus stimulating healthy hair growth.

Dry Hair

Treat over-dry hair and a dry scalp to a pre-shampoo oil pack. Gently heat some olive, almond or jojoba oil in a bowl over a pan of boiling water, apply the warm oil to dry hair and massage in well. Wrap your head in foil or an old towel and sit in the bath for 15 minutes (the steam will help the oil penetrate your hair and scalp). To wash the oil out, apply shampoo directly to the hair without rinsing first, massage, rinse and then shampoo again as normal.

You can combat dryness of the scalp by wrapping your hair in damp towels and sitting in a bath for 15–20 minutes to allow the steam to penetrate the towels.

Greasy Hair

If you have greasy hair take 1 pint (600 ml) of water and add 1 tablespoon (20 ml) of bicarbonate of soda and two beaten eggs. Pour this mixture over hair and massage well into scalp. Leave for 10 minutes, shampoo gently and rinse thoroughly.

Dull Hair

To smooth and brighten dull hair, beat an egg yolk, add it to a small carton of yoghurt and mix thoroughly. Shampoo your hair, then comb the yoghurt and egg mixture through it. Leave it on for 10–15 minutes, then rinse thoroughly with lukewarm water.

If your hair is dull it could be suffering from a build-up of shampoo. Rinse any traces of shampoo away with a weak solution of 2 tablespoons (40 ml) of white vinegar in 3½ pints (2 litres) of water. Use after shampooing and before conditioning.

Damaged Hair

To prevent your hair from becoming dry and damaged, try rubbing a little warm coconut oil into your scalp. Wrap your head in a warm towel and leave for 30 minutes before washing with a mild shampoo.

Split Ends

Prevent split ends by working 'mayonnaise' into clean, dry hair and leaving it on for at least an hour. Either use one of the purer commercial brands that do not contain harmful additives or simply make your own by whisking 1 teaspoon (5 ml) each of oil (vegetable, sunflower or almond) and vinegar together with a large egg until the mixture is well blended and smooth.

Dandruff

To prevent dandruff and to make your hair smell fresh, try a rosemary hair rinse. Put a large handful of rosemary into a pan and cover with water. Simmer for 10–15 minutes and leave to cool. Strain the mixture through a sieve into a jug containing a few drops of wheatgerm or any oil and use as a rinse after you have washed your hair with a very mild shampoo. Finally rinse thoroughly with tepid water.

Stimulating Hair Growth

Stimulate your scalp by using a scalp brush. Never do this when your hair is wet or even damp, but when your hair is completely dry brush deep into scalp at the roots of your hair in a circular motion, beginning from the neck and moving upwards over head. This will encourage strong, healthy growth.

If you want long hair, encourage it to grow by plaiting it, not too tightly at night. Undo the plaits in the morning and you will have gentle waves. When your hair is washed and straight, it will be longer!

Try Japanese-style hair-tugging to promote healthy growth and shine. Bend your head forwards and grasp a hank of hair close to scalp. Tug hard, relax your grip, then tug again. Repeat the procedure three times. Repeat all over scalp, to stimulate new, thicker growth, concentrating on any thinning areas, such as the sides of the forehead.

Hair Loss

Do not worry if some hairs fall out as a result of using a scalp brush. These are dead hairs, which would have fallen out anyway. The average human head loses 100 hairs each day, which corresponds to the hair cycle of growth, loss and regrowth. Stimulating the scalp will encourage stronger and thicker regrowth.

However, you should avoid unnecessary hair fall loss by dis-entangling only when your hair is completely dry, not even damp. Hair is at it's weakest when it is wet and most pliable when it is damp, so trying to pull a comb or brush through it at this stage could result in the loss of otherwise healthy hair. Always use a conditioner, because this helps to prevent tangles from forming.

Severe hair loss may be due to an underlying cause such as anaemia (caused by iron deficiency), an underactive thyroid, hormonal imbalance, stress, the contraceptive pill or prolonged use of medication. If you are at all worried consult a doctor and have a blood test.

Natural Hair Colourants

Gypsies traditionally use strong tea as a hair colourant and tonic. The natural tannin content of tea temporarily darkens grey hair but leaves a natural looking colour. Medium-strength tea will add gloss and sheen to dark hair: save the left-overs from your pot, strain well and use the liquid, cooled, as the last rinse after shampooing. Vinegar has the same effect.

Walnuts can have a slight colouring effect. They were first used to darken and enhance hair colour in Roman times. If you are a brunette, try adding 4oz (100 g) of chopped walnuts to 1 pint (600 ml) of boiling water. Strain, apply the resulting liquid and leave on for 15–20 minutes.

For a natural hair colour, try a herbal rinse to give a soft, subtle effect. Camomile flowers add sheen to blonde hair, nettles are a good tonic for all hair types (but be careful gathering them), and elderberries will add a subtle deep mahogany colour to dark hair. Put a large handful of the appropriate plant into a pan and cover completely with water. Simmer for 20 minutes, strain and leave to cool. After washing your hair with a mild shampoo, use the herbal rinse, then rinse thoroughly with cool water, making sure that no traces of the rinse remain.

Natural Waves

As an alternative to heated appliances, use pipe cleaners to give a natural wavy effect. While your hair is damp, twist strands of it around pipe cleaners, which can be bent back to hold them in place. Leave them in until your hair is dry, then for a wavy, full look, gently comb through.

Instead of reaching for your heated rollers, why not set your hair using old-fashioned rags for an up-to-the-minute look that will not encourage split ends. Wash your hair and leave it to dry naturally. When it is almost dry, take a section of hair and wind it around a rag. When you reach the roots, fold over the ends of the cloth and tie them in a knot. Roll up the rest of your hair in the same way and leave for at least 20 minutes. The longer the rags are left in, the tighter the curls will be. You could even leave them overnight. Unwind the rags and lightly shake out the curls.

Other Tips for Healthy Hair

If at all possible allow your hair to dry naturally, preferably outdoors, particularly if it is sunny, rather than use a hair-drier. After washing towel your hair dry and then use your fingers to shake it gently. Avoid any styling until your hair is completely dry. A hair-drier can be too harsh, can overdry hair and can dry some areas more than others. Besides, drying hair naturally is free!

Keep the use of heated hair appliances to a minimum. Overusing them will damage the cuticle and leave your hair dry and brittle.

Try not to overdo applications of hairspray, mousse or gel. Constantly bombarding your hair with a layer of chemicals weakens it and dulls its texture. Hair needs to breathe to keep the cuticles healthy.

To relieve tension in the scalp and to promote healthy looking hair, try this early morning Indonesian massage technique. Stand with your feet apart and slowly breathe in and out. Gently lean forward from waist, curving your spine, until your head is just below waist level. Keeping your legs straight, gently rap your scalp all over with your knuckles for half a minute. Slowly raise your body and repeat the rapping in an upright position.

Give yourself a daily massage for 5–10 minutes to stimulate circulation, which is vital for healthy hair growth. Using your fingers, work over the surface of the scalp, temples and back of the head, applying pressure in circular movements. Another excellent way of stimulating blood flow to the hair follicles is to practise standing on your head.

Non-greasy handcream can help to reduce static and smooth down flyaway hair. Spread a very small amount in the palms of your hands and stroke it lightly over your hair. It will add a slight sheen, too!

For fresh-smelling hair, add a few drops of your favourite fragrance to the final rinse or leave in conditioner.

Do not wash your hair every day. The lathering agents in many shampoos strip it of natural oils, and some conditioners leave an oily residue, which sits on top of the hair, attracting dirt. Try a milder wash with shampoos that exclude detergents–for example, use one of the frequent-wash shampoos that are widely available now.

Baby powder or fine talcum powder makes a good dry shampoo. Shake a small amount into the roots of the hair, leave for a minute, then brush it out thoroughly.

Avoid brushing dirt and grease back into your hair by washing your brush and comb regularly. Soak them in tepid, soapy water, then rinse well and dry on a folded towel with the bristles facing downwards; never dry over direct heat. Do not soak rubber-cushioned brushes, because the bristles tend to loosen, or wooden-framed brushes, which tend to rot if wet. If your brush is very dirty, dip it in a weak solution of ammonia and water and rinse well.

Always treat your hair with respect. Lock away your heated rollers, tongs and hot brushes for a few weeks and give your hair a well-earned rest. Handle it gently when brushing and combing to avoid tearing and breaking.

EYES

Treatments for Puffy, Sore Eyes

Refresh your eyes by lying down, preferably in a quiet room, for 15 minutes with a slice of either raw potato or cucumber over each eye. Cotton wool pads soaked in witch hazel or in iced water can be used instead. You will notice that your eyes will sparkle and that any puffiness will have disappeared!

Tea has been used as a reviver for less than sparkling eyes for over two centuries! When you have had a late night or a long, hard day, relax with a couple of cooled teabags (the new round ones fit particularly well) over your eyelids for 10 minutes. You're guaranteed to feel instantly revived. It is not just the coolness of the teabag that makes you feel better, the polyphenols and tannin in tea have a mildly astringent and stimulating effect on the skin. Tea also causes skin to tighten slightly, and this helps to reduce puffiness and to remove dark circles.

Natural Ways to Remove Eye Make-up

Cleanse away eye make-up and mascara with a trace of sweet almond oil and cotton wool. Wipe carefully from the nose to the outer eye. Leave a trace of oil on your skin to nourish it. Cotton buds (use one end for each eye) dipped into the oil and wiped gently over eye make-up and mascara will serve the same purpose. Rinse with a gentle toner, preferably one that is alcohol-, colour- and fragrance-free.

Baby oil is an effective eye make-up remover, especially for thick, waterproof mascara. Pour a small amount on to round cotton wool pads and wipe gently over the make-up, using one pad for each eye.

If your eyes are sensitive, dip cotton bud ends directly in the baby oil, remembering to use one end for each eye.

Healthy Eyelashes and Eyebrows

Applying a little petroleum jelly to the root of your lashes each night will encourage healthy growth and make the lashes long and strong. For both day and evening make-up, petroleum jelly can be used to keep your eyebrows in shape and give them a good sheen. Work the jelly into your eyebrows with your fingers, but use only a tiny amount, because too much will look and feel greasy.

Petroleum jelly is also an effective, colourless mascara. Use an old eyelash comb to comb it through your lashes to make them look instantly thicker and longer. It will not clog, cause a sensitive reaction in the eyes nor, because it does not contain colour pigments as mascara does, will it create black marks all over your eyes when you cry!

Eyelash curlers obviate the need for mascara. However, if you have fair hair you might want to consider having your lashes dyed dark brown, which is far cheaper in the long run and is kinder to your eyes. However, do not attempt to dye your lashes yourself with hair dye. It is far better to seek professional help.

One way in which you can avoid expensive beauty treatments is by simply brushing your eyebrows into shape every night. Take an eyebrow brush (an old, soft toothbrush will do) and guide the eyebrows into the shape you want. Smooth a little petroleum jelly on to stubborn hairs to keep them in shape.

HANDS

Your hands are on show to the world, so make sure that you try these simple but effective treatments for soft, supple hands.

Once a week, thoroughly moisturize your hands with an effective handcream and put on a pair of close-fitting, but not too tight cotton gloves. Leave them on for as long as possible, preferably overnight. The perspiration from your hands will blend with the cream to soften the skin thoroughly. This treatment will also help to reduce any prominent veins on the hands.

Keep your fingers slim and your hands soft by brushing the surface of hands and fingers with a cushioned brush – a hairbrush with cushioned balls on the spikes is ideal – towards the heart. This also improves circulation and helps to prevent unsightly raised veins.

Hand Workout

Hands need exercise, too, to keep them soft and slim and to keep the joints functioning smoothly. Try the following easy exercises daily, and you will become more nimble fingered!

For a warm-up, form your hands into fist shapes (Fig. 2a), hold for a few seconds and then release. Repeat ten times. Next join your hands together, pressing the palms flat against each other with your fingers straight as if you were praying (Fig. 2b). Fold over the fingers of one hand into the spaces between fingers of the other hand, making sure that they are folded over completely (Fig. 2c). Press your fingers as hard as possible for a few seconds and release. Repeat ten times. Finally, separate your hands and stretch out your fingers as far as possible (Fig. 2d); then relax. Repeat ten times. Rest and relax your hands and fingers for a few minutes.

Now you are ready to start the elastic band exercises. Put one end of a thick elastic band over the joint of the thumb, and the other end over the last joint of the first finger. Stretch the elastic band as far as it will go, relax and repeat ten times. Repeat the exercise separately with each of the second, third, and fourth fingers on both hands. Rest for a few minutes, then place the elastic band over the middle of thumb and all fingers to form a circle. Stretch the elastic band as far as possible and relax. Repeat ten times. These exercises are useful for keyboard users to prevent repetitive strain injury, and they will help those who suffer from rheumatism and arthritis.

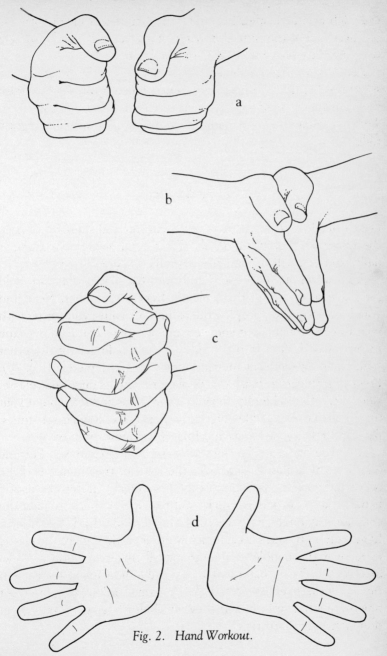

Fig. 2.   Hand Workout.

Dry Hands

Dry hands need intensive treatments. Mix 1 teaspoon (5 ml) of honey with a little vegetable, almond or olive oil and massage the lotion directly on to your hands, leaving it for as long as possible before rinsing with a soap-free cleanser.

To exfoliate dead skin from the hands, blend some granulated sugar with a little oil (whichever type is handy) and rub well in. Rinse to reveal soft, new, gentle skin. This treatment also evens out the skin tone. Another way of achieving exfoliation is by moving a body brush loaded with a soap-free cleanser over your hands, including the palms. Rinse with cold water. This also improves circulation and speeds up skin renewal.

Help to make cracked, dry hands soft and supple by keeping a bottle of sweet almond oil next to the wash-basin. Add a few drops of oil to the warm water every time you wash your hands.

Once a week, try this hand treatment to pamper and soften your hands. Make a simple hand lotion by mixing 2 teaspoons (10 ml) of olive oil with 1 teaspoon (5 ml) of liquid honey. You can also add a drop of your favourite perfume or aromatherapy oil. Massage the mixture well into the hands, leave for a few minutes then wash off with warm, soapy water or a gentle shower gel.

Slough off dry, discoloured skin with a gentle scrub made from 1 tablespoon (20 ml) each of sunflower oil and salt mixed together well. Rub on to your skin and rinse with warm, soapy water or a gentle shower gel.

If you enjoy gardening but your hands suffer, smooth on this cream under your work gloves. Mix together 1 dessertspoon (10 ml) of almond oil and an equal amount of fuller's earth with two egg yolks. Smooth this on to your hands and put on your gloves. When you have finished gardening rinse away the lotion and your hands will have had a wonderful treatment while you have been working hard.

Split Nails

Prevent nails from splitting and chipping by encouraging healthy nail growth with an oil bath. Gently warm some almond oil, then soak your fingertips in the oil for about 10 minutes. Take time to push cuticles back with a cotton bud after the soaking.

Protect your nails at all times from the damaging effects of gardening, housework, DIY and especially washing-up. Rubber gloves keep out the wet but wearing them too much actually softens the nails you are trying to strengthen. A good idea is to wear a pair of fine cotton gloves, which are available from chemists, under the rubber ones.

Natural Manicure

For a quick home manicure, try the following. Clean off the old nail polish with plenty of remover. Shape your nails with an emery board, filing from side to centre in long, easy strokes. Give your hands a thorough wash, scrubbing your nails with lots of soapy water. Dry your hands carefully and work in lots of handcream, massaging the nail bed (see below). Then gently push back the cuticles with a cotton bud. Rinse away any traces of handcream and dry.

To encourage blood flow and thus growth, massage each nail bed for about a minute every evening with just a little sweet almond oil. The nail bed, where all the growth occurs, is just below the skin's surface immediately next to the cuticle.

Almond oil is an excellent nail and cuticle conditioner. Simply work a little oil into each nail plate and leave for about 10 minutes before washing away. It will leave your nails looking and feeling wonderfully healthy. Alternatively, to encourage strong and healthy growth, rub petroleum jelly into your nails and nail bed at night. Wipe off any excess.

To achieve salon-effect 'French polish' nails, gently massage petroleum jelly into the nail and nail bed. Tissue off by gently rubbing with a soft tissue. For added shine, give a quick rub over with a nail buffer. This treatment is good for nails with or without nail polish.

For the natural look of a French manicure, try the following: make sure your nails are clean and neatly filed and that all old nail enamel has been removed. If your nails are discoloured, lighten them with a cotton bud dipped in white wine vinegar. Paint on a clear base coat, allow it to dry and put on a light coat of white pearl polish. Leave to dry, then apply one coat of pale pink polish, finishing off with a clear top coat to add shine.

LIPS

Petroleum jelly is essential for smooth, well-defined lips. It is the ideal colourless lip-gloss, which you can apply directly to your lips with your fingers or you can use a lip-brush or a cotton bud. Petroleum jelly can be used on its own or with lipstick. If you apply it before lipstick you will create a subtle sheen; applied on top of lipstick it will give a glamorous gloss. Applying petroleum jelly to your lips every night will condition them and help to avoid wrinkles.

Cold Sores

Lemon juice is said to prevent cold sores. Citric acid quickly kills bacteria, making it a natural cleanser for grimy skin, and it would be well worth rubbing a slice of lemon over your lips if you get that itchy, pre-cold sore feeling.

Natural Gloss

If one of your lips is darker than the other – the top lip is usually darker than the bottom lip – rub a slice of lemon over your top lip every day and rinse with cold water. This treatment also smoothes lips, so you may want to rub the lemon over both lips, but pay greater attention to the upper lip to make the colours even. Cocoa butter also has a smoothing effect on lips. Blend it in with your fingers, leaving it on overnight for maximum benefit.

If you want to give your lips a natural shade of red, cut a strawberry in half, using half for each lip. Rub the end of the strawberry over your lip and rinse with warm water. If you do not have any strawberries, crushed raspberries or redcurrants can also be used.

Smooth on moisturizer or night cream as a base either before make-up, to prevent lipstick leaving stains on your lips, or at night, to condition and soften, especially in cold weather.

Chapped Lips

Honey is an excellent natural moisturizer. Simply rub it into your lips whenever they are sore or chapped. Leave it on for as long as possible.

Lined Lips

If your lips have lines, try exfoliation to diminish them. Again, you can use sugar mixed with oil or scrubs, which should be rubbed on to your lips and rinsed off with warm water.

Lip Exercises

Lips need exercise just like any other muscles. Look under facial exercises (see page 56) or simply stretch your lips by forming a wide smile and relax. Repeat five times. Curl your lips over your teeth and join your top and bottom teeth together. Relax. Repeat five times. Join your lips together and push forward as far as you can. Relax and repeat five times.

These exercises should help to prevent lines forming around your lips and make your lips fuller, thus preventing lipstick from 'feathering'.

TEETH

Stained Teeth

Tackle everyday stains on your teeth – those caused by tobacco and wine, for example – by brushing with bicarbonate of soda. Dip a wet toothbrush into the powder to coat it and then brush directly on to your teeth, paying particular attention to those at the front. Rinse or brush as normal afterwards. If the stains are really stubborn, try adding lemon juice as well as the soda to the toothbrush. Brush as before.

An effective mouthwash can be made from 2 teaspoons (10 ml) of salt in a glass of warm water. This will also strengthen your gums. Gargle thoroughly with the salted water, making sure that the back teeth have been reached. Add a dash of lemon juice to the water to brighten yellow teeth. The salt will neutralize any acid remaining on the teeth even after brushing, thus controlling the build up of plaque, the cause of tooth decay and gum disease. Do this in the morning and last thing at night for strong teeth and healthy gums.

If you have had something very sugary to eat and cannot brush your teeth between meals, eat some salted peanuts. Again, the salt will neutralize the sugary acid. Eating cheese, with its high calcium content, will help to keep your teeth strong.

Hold 1 teaspoon (5 ml) of sunflower oil in your mouth for 15 minutes to clean your teeth. Rinse and brush thoroughly afterwards.

Brushing alone is not enough to keep your teeth and gums healthy. Floss with unwaxed floss at least once a day, especially at night. Wind a length around your fingers and pass it gently between two teeth, working it up into the gum crevices and down to the biting surface. Pull gently against one side of the teeth and then the other. Do not tug at the gentle gums; always treat them with the respect they deserve.

Change your toothbrush at least every three months. When you choose a brush, take the shape of your teeth into account; if your teeth are small, you will be able to clean them better with a small tooth-brush. Try not to brush too hard, as this can lead to receding gums and possible disease. Be gentle but thorough.

Fresh Breath

An infusion of camomile tea will make sure that your breath is fresh. When it is cool, it is a delicious, economical mouthwash, much better than the expensive, purchased mouthwashes, which can be too strong and which can sometimes contain alcohol as well as artificial colours.

A drop of peppermint oil added to warm water makes an instant mouth freshener.

NECK

The skin on the neck is the first to show the signs of ageing, so pay especial attention here. The skin on the neck is very fine, and it is wise, therefore, to avoid heavy creams or moisturizers in this delicate area, because they could accentuate lines and stretch the skin, making the neck muscles sag even further.

Use only light oils on the neck; evening primrose oil is very good for the delicate skin on the neck, but any good oil will do the trick, even vegetable oil or olive oil. Sweet almond oil is inexpensive and effective. Massage in the oil of your choice, preferably at night so that the oil can penetrate into the skin for maximum benefit.

Always try to apply a moisturizer before you go out, because the skin in the neck area has very few sebaceous glands and it can get dry very easily. You will probably have noticed that you get hardly any blemishes on the neck, and this lack of sebaceous glands is the reason. If your neck looks too shiny after applying oil, gently tissue off the excess with a facial tissue.

Exfoliate gently everyday. You should, ideally, do this at night, when the skin repairs itself, to allow the skin to speed up its renewal process, dislodge dead cells and smooth out lines. This area responds to, and needs, exfoliation more than any other area – even more than the face. The emphasis is on being gentle. Harsh exfoliation in this delicate area can cause redness. Use a soft facial brush with a mild soap and warm water or massage with ground oatmeal.

The exercises for the neck, jaw and chin in the facial exercises section (see pages 57–59) will improve the tone and condition of the skin and will help to smooth out any surplus lines.

Once a week, use a moisturizing mask. Try mixing 1 tablespoon (20 ml) of honey with 2 tablespoons (40 ml) of almond oil. Gently brush the lotion on to the neck with a soft brush (a pastry brush will do). Leave on for 30 minutes and rinse with warm water. Your skin will feel soft and smooth.

FEET

Your feet will reveal the first signs of neglect, but a little care will go a long way. While you are having a bath or shower wet your loofah or body brush with warm water and soap or shower gel. Vigorously rub all over your feet with the loofah or brush, paying particular attention to the soles and to any corns. Rinse with warm water, and dry thoroughly.

To soften your feet, try this treatment once a week. Thoroughly moisturize your feet with body cream or lotion, put on some closely fitting, but not too tight, cotton socks and leave them on for as long as possible, preferably overnight. When you remove the socks, the sweat from your feet will have blended with the cream to soften your feet miraculously! Wash afterwards with a mild soap or shower gel.

If you have had a hard day, soothe tired feet by putting some warm, salted water into a large bowl. Add about twenty large marbles and move your feet around over the marbles. The marbles will have a relaxing, massaging effect.

If you do not want to wet your feet, try gliding them backwards and forwards over a rolling pin. This provides a gentle, soothing action, particularly for the in-step. You could also try this action with your feet immersed in water if you preferred.

Soothe away aching feet with a 10-minute soak in a warm footbath, with a few drops of lavender oil or some bath crystals added. Then plunge your feet into cold water before drying them thoroughly. A quick rub down with lemon juice will also help to revive tired, sore feet. Shopper's blisters can be eased by dusting with cornflour, which helps to soothe and heal, too.

To relieve your feet after a hard day and to recirculate blood that has settled in feet and lower legs, lie on the floor near a wall. Raise your legs over your head. Resting your feet on the wall, hold them there for 2 minutes or as long as required to improve blood circulation. If your feet are tired and swollen from too much standing, stimulate the circulation by dipping them alternately in a basin of hot water, then in to one of cold water; the more extreme the temperatures, the better. Dry gently.

Keep your ankles supple with this easy exercise. Sit with your legs stretched out in front of you and point a dozen imaginary circles with the toes of each foot, turning first in a clockwise direction and then in the opposite direction.

Remove old nail polish with an oily remover and wash your feet in warm, soapy water to get rid of stubborn dirt. Clip toe nails straight across; avoid cutting corners at an angle to prevent ingrowing nails. Use a pumice stone to remove excess dry skin from soles and heels. Do not rub too vigorously – regular, light use is best.

4

Exercises for Face and Body

FACIAL EXERCISES

Most facial expressions do not use the muscles that keep contours youthful, and they can actually encourage wrinkles. Facial exercises, on the other hand, concentrate on specific, often lazy and unused muscles. You can build up facial muscles as you can those of your body, and, just as with other parts of your body, well-toned muscles mean firmer contours. Because the muscles are connected to the skin, you can keep the skin of your face well supported for longer.

Relieving Tension

To soothe away tension and prevent premature wrinkles, try the following Chinese exercises.

Warm your hands by rubbing them briskly together. Place the middle fingers of each hand over your eyelids, just below the brow bone, and apply gentle pressure. Repeat three times.

Place the fingers of both hands horizontally and flat against your forehead. Press firmly against the bone, pulling the skin upwards and outwards very slightly; at the same time, move your eyebrows down and slowly close your eyes tight until you feel your eyes and your forehead pulling in opposite directions. Use your little fingers to pull between your brows to prevent frown lines. Relax and repeat three times.

To tone jaw muscles, which can accumulate tension in your face, first locate the muscles by placing your fingers at the sides of your face and closing and opening your mouth a few times. Put your forefingers into the hollows at the hinges of your jaw. Pressing down, make smooth rotating movements with your fingertips for 30 seconds.

Rub the palms of your hands briskly up and down your cheeks. With your middle fingers, stroke from the centre of the forehead towards the temples, smoothing away frown lines. Using your fingertips and in decreasing circles, massage away tension. Use your eyes, nose, cheeks, jaw and mouth to pull as many faces as possible.

Preventing Lines and Wrinkles

To prevent lines from forming around your nose and mouth, slightly curl your upper lip around your top teeth and your lower lip around your bottom teeth. Press your lips firmly together and blow as hard as you can, keeping your mouth closed, for a count of six. Relax and repeat three times.

Form your mouth into an O shape, pushing your jaw and upper lip forwards. Slightly curl your upper lip over your top teeth, hold for a count of six, then relax. Repeat the exercise but with your head tilted back. Then turn your head to the right, and repeat the O movement. Do exactly the same with your head turned to the left. Repeat the entire sequence three times.

To tone up your cheek muscles, fill your mouth with water – it's pressure that does the work – and hold it there for as long as possible. Then relax.

For strong cheek and chin muscles, smile with your mouth closed, raising your cheeks and the corners of your lips up towards your eyes. Hold for a count of six, then, in the same position, jut your jaw forwards and hold this position for a count of six. Relax, then grin, this time with your mouth slightly open and stretching the corners of your mouth out to the sides. Count to six, then, in the same position, jut your jaw forwards and count to six. Relax. Repeat the entire exercise three times.

To help prevent a double chin from developing, jut out your chin and, using the back of the fingers of each hand, gently tap upwards for a stimulating massage. Use a firm, bouncy motion, drumming, but not slapping too hard, against the skin with each hand alternately for 30 seconds.

To strengthen your neck muscles, purse your lips together and place your forefingers on your neck, one each side of your windpipe. Massage smoothly, up and down, with firm, gentle strokes, for 30 seconds.

Exercises for Your Eyes

Prevent 'crow's feet' from developing by pressing the middle and third fingers horizontally at the corner of your eyes. Close your eyes slowly, using the muscles under the eyes. Count to six and repeat three times.

The formation of droopy skin above the eyes can be prevented by placing your index fingers under your eyebrows. Press on the bone and lift upwards slightly, at the same time closing your lids tightly. When you feel a slight pull on the skin, count to six. Relax, open your eyes and repeat three times.

To avoid eye fatigue, press firmly for a second at the pressure point on the bridge of your nose. Repeat five times.

Ease eyestrain by looking up, then down, then to the far right and the far left. Look from top right diagonally to bottom left, and from top left to bottom right. Look up, then circle your eyes from the side in a clockwise direction. Then circle in an anti-clockwise direction. Hold your thumb about 12 in (30 cm) from your eyes, focus on imaginary walls behind and in front of your thumb. (Fig. 3.) End by 'palming'

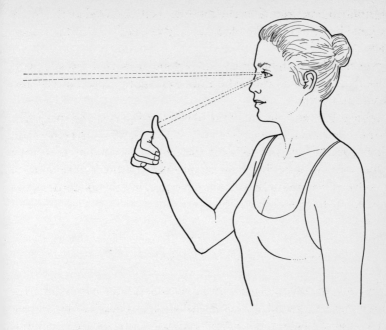

Fig. 3. Ease eyestrain by holding your thumb about 12 in (30 cm) from your eyes and focusing on imaginary walls, one in front of your thumb, the other behind it.

eyes: rub your palms together until they are warm, then cup your hands over closed eyes. The warmth and darkness will combine to relax your eyes.

BODY EXERCISES

Posture

Your mother will probably have advised you to 'stand tall', and she was right. You can tell a lot about a person who slouches: it usually shows that they have a low opinion of themselves. Good posture is not just about self-esteem, however; it is essential to prevent problems with the back, ribs and even the lungs, and while bad posture can create bulges where there should not be any, good posture will make you look 5 lb (more than 2 kg) slimmer instantly!

Bad posture can result in the following unnecessary problems: tension around the neck and shoulders; lines on the neck become more pronounced; difficulties arise with the chest and breathing; the breasts fall in and droop; the stomach sticks out. All these are avoidable.

Try these tips for good posture. Straighten your neck upwards, but do not stretch it. Relax your shoulders, taking them back if you have a tendency to slouch inwards; the outside of the shoulders should be straight, not bent inwards towards the chest. Hold your stomach in by breathing in; a relaxed stomach will simply flop out.

The buttocks should not stick out. If they do, try to bring your hips inwards, to align with your waist. The old technique of walking with a book on the head is effective, or you could try hanging from the door jamb or standing straight against a wall. Do not overstraighten, however, but follow the spine's natural shape.

Your spine and neck should lengthen upwards, with your head balanced lightly on the top of the spine. When you consider that your head weighs in the region of 14 lb (6 kg), you will appreciate that if it is pushed forward, it will strain the neck and shoulder muscles, forcing your whole body to compensate for the imbalance. Relax your chest, shoulders and upper back; do not push your shoulders upwards or forwards.

Develop strength and stability through your pelvis, legs and feet, allowing them to come into natural balance and line and sending their weight, through your legs and feet, towards the floor. Constantly remind yourself to relax and to align your posture. Arrange your home, desk and work place so that you can avoid unnecessary twists and turns. Always bend and lift correctly, using your leg muscles and flexing at the knees and hips while you keep your back straight.

At the end of a busy day lie down flat on the floor for 10 minutes, allowing your weight to 'drop' towards the ground. Breathe slowly and deeply to dispel stress and tension. Change your mood by applying the principle of posture balance. Think length, width and support in your body, and you will feel much better for it. Massage (see Chapter

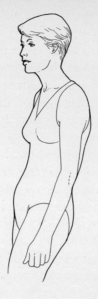

Fig. 4(a). A poor, slumped posture.

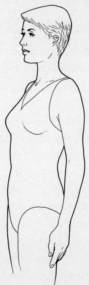

Fig. 4(b). See the difference that standing tall and keeping the spine erect can make.

5) can be beneficial by helping to break down muscular tension and by rebalancing and realigning posture.

The Alexander Technique (see Further Reading, page 115) re-educates you in movement, focusing on the release and alignment of the spine, neck and head.

Relieving Tension

To relieve tension and boost your energy levels try this yoga exercise. Stand with your feet 18 in (45 cm) apart, and your arms hanging loosely at your sides. Beginning with your head, allow your body to relax forwards from the waist. Let your head and arms hang limply. Without straining, allow your body to bend further forwards until it is as low as feels comfortable (see Fig. 5). Hold this position for a count of ten. Slowly straighten up, remaining relaxed, with your head being raised last.

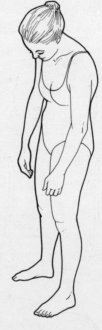

Fig. 5. Let your whole body go limp.

Relieve shoulder tension by sitting with your back straight and your arms and hands relaxed. Inhale through your nose and keep your mouth closed. Rotate your shoulders backwards, raising them to your ears, while you hold your breath, count to five, then slowly exhale, relaxing your neck and bringing your shoulders forward to their normal position. Take a short rest, then repeat. Whenever you feel tension in your shoulders, do this sequence up to six times (Fig. 6).

Ease migraine, headaches and period pains by adopting a relaxation pose known as 'the corpse'. Lie on your back on the floor with your legs slightly apart and your arms apart from your sides with the palms upwards. Practise deep abdominal breathing, filling your abdomen like a balloon as you inhale and letting it go as you exhale. Feel yourself relaxing more and more with each exhalation. Do this for at least 5 minutes. It relieves stress and lowers the pulse rate.

The yoga 'complete breath' is one of the easiest ways to begin learning to use your lungs efficiently and is very helpful to those suffering from respiratory ailments such as asthma, bronchitis and so forth.

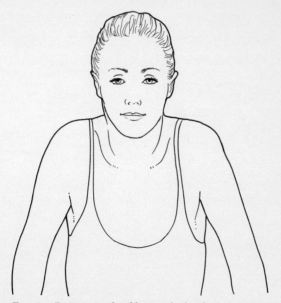

Fig. 6. Raise your shoulders to the level of your ears.

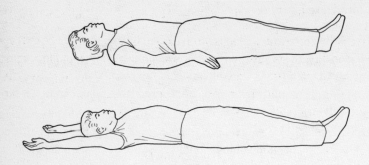

Fig. 7. The 'complete breath'.

Lie on a rug on the floor, or ground if outside, with your arms at your sides, several centimetres away from your body, palms face down (Fig. 7).

Close your eyes and inhale through your nose very slowly. Expand your abdomen slightly, then pull the air up into the rib-cage, and then your chest. Hold for a few seconds.

Now breathe out slowly through your nose in a smooth continuous flow until the abdomen is drawn in and the rib-cage and chest are relaxed. Hold for a few seconds before repeating two or three times.

Now breathe in slowly and gradually raise your arms overhead in time with the inhalation until the backs of your hands touch the floor.

Hold your breath for ten seconds.

Slowly breathe out as you bring your arms back down to your sides. Repeat two or three times.

A similar technique will allow you to achieve complete relaxation of your mind and body. Unplug the phone and lie down slowly, flat on your back, with your legs together and your arms at your sides. Allow your feet to part as you relax your leg and feet muscles. With your palms upwards, let your arms go limp. Tilt your head back by raising your chin and close your eyes. Relax all your facial muscles, allowing your mouth to drop open. Concentrate on your breathing and let it slow down. If your attention wanders, gently guide it back to your breathing. Even a few minutes in this position gives complete relaxation. Get up very slowly.

To ease indigestion, which is often caused by tension, stand with your back and head straight, with your arms relaxed by your side. Pull in your stomach muscles and take a very deep breath, count to five, then slowly breathe out and relax the upper part of the body. Breathe normally, then repeat five times.

Toning Muscles

Try some simple yoga exercises to tone up your body. The system of deep abdominal breathing in yoga both releases physical and mental tension and increases energy.

To improve your circulation try these exercises first thing in the morning. Stand up straight and slowly rotate your shoulders backwards, first one at a time, then together. Slowly bend your neck, first to one side, then to the other so that you feel a gentle stretch in your neck. With your hands on your hips, bend to each side from the waist, holding the position for a few seconds. Keeping your hands on your hips and with your feet apart, bend at the knees, then stretch up on to your toes. Repeat five times.

Working out encourages the production of a hormone called beta-endorphin, which helps to combat stress and gives you a good feeling. Working out also helps you burn up calories!

Try these simple, fun exercises first thing in the morning to get you going.

Stand as straight as possible, but with back as comfortable as possible. Now jump, stretching out your arms and legs as you do so (Fig. 8). Return to an upright position and repeat the exercise ten times.

To tone the muscles of your hips and waist, stretch out your arms slightly from the straight position. Keep your legs together, bend your

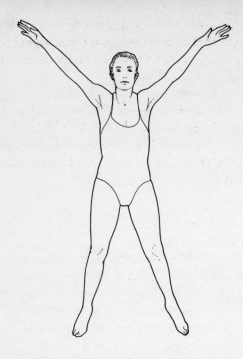

Fig. 8. Jump in the air, stretching out your arms and legs as you rise.

knees slightly and move your feet to the left. Now, jumping off the ground, perform a semicircle movement so that your feet are now to your immediate right. Do this ten times.

Running on the spot is an excellent form of exercise, which you can even do while you watch television. If possible, open a nearby

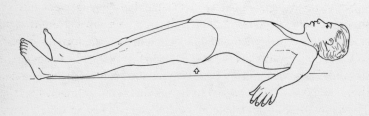

Fig. 9. Use only the muscles in your buttocks to lift your body from the floor.

window so that you can gain the full benefit of your increased inhalation and exhalation. Then, from the standing position, bend down as far as you can with knees together, then jump up as far as you can. Try this ten times.

After some gentle aerobic exercises you may want to relax by lying down flat on the floor for 5 minutes. While you relax, you can tighten your buttocks, and use your buttock muscles to lift your body gently off the floor (Fig. 9). Hold for a few seconds, then relax. Repeat ten times or more daily.

SWIMMING EXERCISES

Swimming is considered to be the best all-round exercise there is, and swimming once or twice a week will show immediate benefits to your body and well-being. Although swimming does use all parts of the body, here are a few exercises that concentrate on specific, stubborn areas.

The weight of the water will make you use greater force to move, thereby making the exercises more effective. Water is also a safer medium than air; it absorbs any shocks and tends to cushion against injuries, and you are less likely to suffer the cramps and injuries often associated with other kinds of exercise.

Warm-Up Exercises

Before you begin, try these easy, gentle, warm-up exercises, which will gently flex your joints and muscles.

Stand up straight in the pool so that the water comes up to your shoulders and keep your legs straight and your arms straight at your sides. Now, keeping them straight, gently bring your arms up in a circle so that they are just below water level (Fig. 10). Still keeping them straight, bring your arms forwards in front of you, again in a circle, so that your hands meet (keep your hands flat and your fingers together). Then reverse these movements so that you reach your initial starting position. Repeat the exercise ten times. This is a good warm-up exercise for the upper body, shoulders, arms and waist (Fig. 11).

67

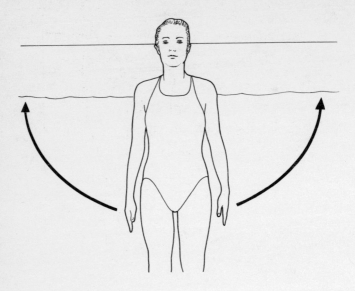

Fig. 10.   *Keeping your arms straight, raise them from your sides until they are just below water level.*

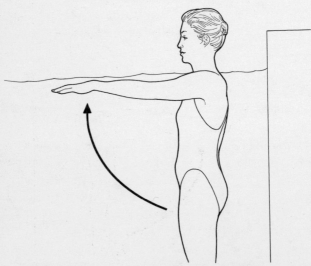

Fig. 11.   *Still with straight arms and keeping them parallel to the water's surface, move them so that they are outstretched in front of you.*

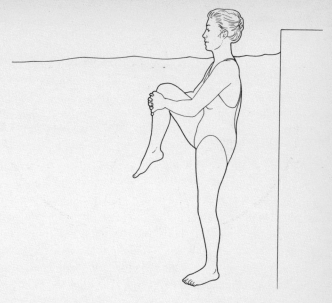

Fig. 12. *Raise your knee as high in the water as you can.*

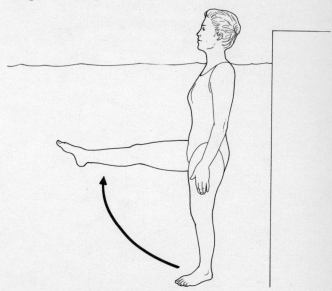

Fig. 13. *Straighten your leg, remembering to point your toes and to keep your leg as high in the water as you can.*

69

Now try these warm-ups for the lower body, thighs and legs. Adopt the initial starting position again, but then, with both arms holding on to your left knee, gently raise it as far as it will go, preferably above waist level. Stand up straight again and repeat the exercise with your right knee. Repeat ten times with each knee (Fig. 12).

Next, with your hands on your waist, bring up your left knee and push your leg out in front of you so that it is straight. Move your straight leg in a circle, then bring it down to standing position again. Do the same with your right leg, repeating the movement ten times with each leg (Fig. 13).

Raise your left arm out to the side so that it is parallel with, and just below, water level. Keeping your body and your legs straight, gently move your left leg in a circle, raising it to the left to try to touch your hand with your toes. Don't worry if you can't do this; reach as far as you can, without overstretching your muscles. Bring your leg back down so that you are in the standing position again and repeat the procedure with your right leg. Do this exercise ten times for each leg (Fig. 14).

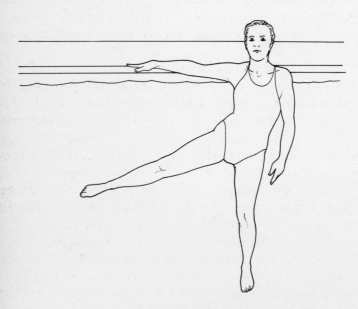

Fig. 14. *Standing upright, raise your leg to the side as far as you can, keeping it as straight as possible.*

Gently relax your neck. Stand straight up again and gently bend your head forwards so that your chin touches your chest. Then move your head back as far as it will go, but only go as far as you feel comfortable. Never overstrain your neck. Then move your head to the left as far as it will go and again to the right (Fig. 15). Repeat each movement five times.

Finally, an exercise that will help you develop your ability to hold your breath underwater. Keeping your body straight, bend your knees so that you are gradually immersed in the water (Fig. 16). Hold the position for a few seconds and quickly come up again. Repeat five times.

Main Exercises

When you have completed the initial warm-up routine in the water, you will feel sufficiently confident to do the main exercises. Put in as much effort as you can but do not overdo it. Increase the amount of energy you put into the exercises as you become more familiar with them.

To do the first exercise you should find a point in the pool where the water level is up to your neck when you are standing upright. This simple exercise will trim your waist, tighten your hips and strengthen your thighs.

Rest your head against the bar and stretch out your arms, keeping them straight along the bar and with your hands holding on to the bar. Stand still with your legs straight. Slowly raise your left leg to the side, and, with your toes pointed, try to touch the bar or your left hand. Reach as far as you can to the left, being careful not to overstretch. Hold your leg in position for a few seconds then lower it to the floor of the pool and resume an upright position. Do the same with your right leg. Repeat the exercise ten times for each leg.

Next, still with your arms parallel to the bar and from an initial standing position with your legs together, bend your knees and move your body round to the left. Your knees should be at waist height and

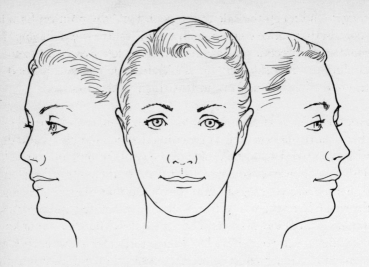

Fig. 15.   To keep your neck supple, turn your head to the left, then the right, as far as you can.

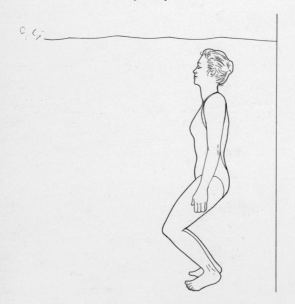

Fig. 16.   Bend your knees slowly so that you are gradually submerged; hold your breath for as long as you can before re-surfacing.

they should touch the side of the pool. Hold the position for a few seconds, then move your knees in a semicircle to the right (Fig. 17). Hold for a few seconds and again circle to the left. Repeat the exercise, circling to each side ten times. Again, this exercise is good for trimming the waist and firming the thighs and buttocks.

Another exercise that is useful for firming thighs and buttocks but that is particularly good for tightening stomach muscles is also done while you stand against the side of the pool, holding on to the bar. This time, however, you can either bend your elbows or keep them straight. Raise your legs in front of you, so that they are floating in the water. Keep them together, with the toes pointed. Relax for a few minutes as your legs float gently on the water. Then bend your knees until they touch your chest. Hold the position for a few seconds and then, with as much effort as you can, push your feet forwards so that your legs are straight, parallel to the surface of the water, with your toes pointed. Hold the position for a few seconds. Repeat the exercise twenty times.

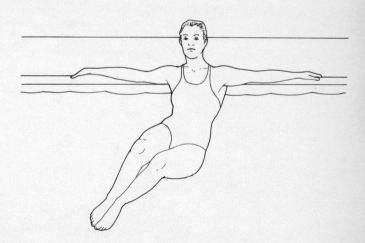

Fig. 17. *Raise your knees and turn your body, first to one side, then to the other.*

The following exercise benefits the upper body, including the bust, arms, shoulders and neck. It will also help to reduce a double chin! It is almost the same as sit-ups, but in the water.

Stand facing the bar, with your legs together and straight. Bend your elbows and hold on to the bar. Now lift your body so that your chin reaches over the top of the bar. Hold for a few seconds, then lower yourself to the standing position.

Repeat at least twenty times, increasing the number each time you do the exercise.

If you find the last exercise difficult, try this gentler version. This will still build strength in the upper body and reduces flabby arms.

Holding on to the bar with your hands, float on your front, with your arms and legs stretched out straight. Bend your elbows and pull yourself towards the bar until your head touches it. Then push yourself back to the starting position. Repeat twenty times.

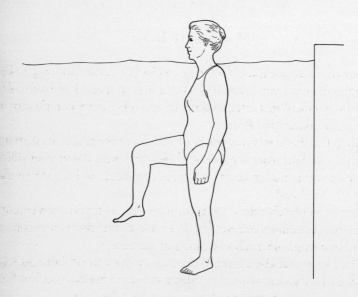

Fig. 18. Walking with water up to your neck is excellent exercise – and harder than it sounds.

Exercises for Face and Body

Walking in Water

During the exercises you may like to try walking in water! This may sound strange, but it really is more effective than ordinary walking.

For the best results, find the point in the pool where the water level reaches your neck. If you are a beginner and feel uncomfortable, go further towards the shallow end until the water just covers your shoulders. It is important that the water should cover your body because it will support your limbs while at the same time making your muscles work harder as you move against it.

Walk from one side of the pool straight across to the other side. This is more difficult than it sounds because the water will exert pressure against you, and you will have to work quite hard. Put in as much effort as you can making sure that you raise your knees to your waist and move your arms (Fig. 18). Walk about 55 yards (50 metres) in all.

Relaxation Technique

When you have completed all the exercises described above, try this relaxing float to cool down. If you are a beginner and have difficulty floating, you will feel safer, and be able to relax more completely, if you use armbands and floats.

Go to the shallow end of the pool and float flat on your back, with your legs straight, your toes pointed and your arms flat at your sides. You may want to keep the float under your back, or hold on to the bar with one hand.

Float, completely relaxed, for 5 minutes, limiting your movements to the bare minimum necessary to keep afloat. Imagine you are on an island in a tropical paradise, basking in the sun.

You can repeat the exercise, floating on your front, but you will find it easier if your arms are stretched together in front of you, holding on to the bar if you need to. Again, float for 5 minutes.

Floating allows all your muscles to rest, because it is the soothing water, and not muscle exertion, that is holding you up.

5

Relaxing, Natural Treatments

A brief outline of some useful complementary therapies follows, which can really work wonders for your health and general well-being, helping you to relax as well as offering treatment for some specific conditions.

FINDING A THERAPIST

A qualified therapist can vastly improve your overall well-being but it is important to bear in mind that they are usually not qualified medical practitioners. Always go to a therapist recommended by a reputable professional association such as those listed under Useful Addresses (see page 115).

You should also bear the following points in mind. A therapist, if not medically qualified, should not offer medical diagnoses. During the first session, the therapist should take a detailed medical case history and ask you what other medication you are taking and for details of past ailments. Your therapist should work with your doctor and refer you to your doctor if he or she can treat you more appropriately. The therapist should not state that the therapy alone is sufficient to treat you.

Your therapist should not pretend to know everything or try to cure or heal you if you are suffering from a serious, life-threatening illness such as cancer. The therapist should not say that there is a miracle cure and should advise you to stop if the treatments are not successful or have reached their limit.

MASSAGE

Although an all-over body massage will, of course, require a practitioner, there are some massage treatments – on your feet and face, for example – that you can carry out yourself, and a simple back massage can be given by a partner or friend.

Foot Massage

Daily foot massage is considered an essential in Far Eastern countries. It is believed to boost the body's immune system, and it also, of course, keeps the feet flexible and the ankles slim. Sit with your legs crossed. Grasp a foot in both hands and knead the arch with your thumbs. Massage the sole and sides of the foot with your thumbs and fingertips. Gently bend each toe. Squeeze your foot rhythmically, alternating the pressure exerted by each hand. Stroke your foot, from toe to ankle and back. Grasp the front of your foot with both hands and knead the sole and arch again. Flex your toes to and fro gently and rotate each one. Place your foot flat on the floor and stroke it towards the toes. Repeat with the other foot (Fig. 19).

You can also try 20 minutes of energizing 'Do-In' massage, an oriental form of self-massage that uses light tapping movements to stimulate sleepy nerve endings and to raise energy levels. Sit on the floor and gently tap the sole of each foot with your knuckles. Tap up and down each leg, from ankle to hip, continuing over the body and along each arm. Finish with light tapping movements over the scalp, shoulders and neck.

Lymphatic Drainage Massage

The technique of Lymphatic drainage massage helps to flush away impurities from the face. With firm, sweeping movements, run your fingertips around both eye sockets and back across the cheeks. Next take the fingers out from the chin along each side of the jawline. Repeat fifteen times (Fig. 20).

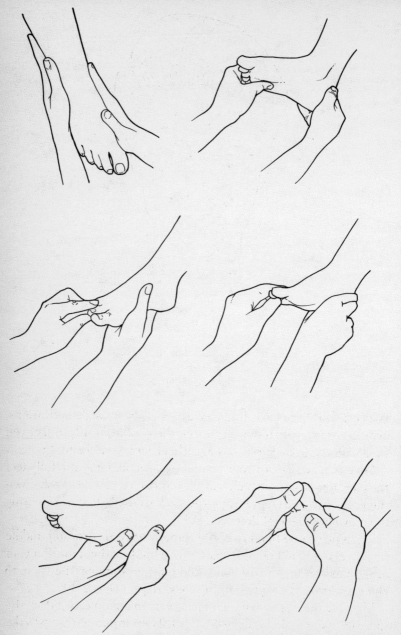

Fig. 19. Foot massage sequence.

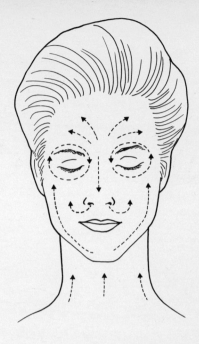

Fig. 20. *Lymphatic drainage massage.*

Back Massage

Be gentle with your back. If you have back problems or complications, avoid massage, which may aggravate the condition. If you feel you would benefit from gentle massage, check with your doctor first.

Give this massage to your partner or a friend. First, carefully feel the back for tensions, which will show up as red patches. Push down the back with both hands from the neck to the buttocks, repeating the movement several times (Fig. 21a).

Then place one hand over the spine, with your first and middle fingers, about ½ in (12 mm) apart, on each side of the spine. Put your other hand on top of this hand, and press, pushing up the spine to clear any blocked channels in the back. Repeat (Fig. 21b).

Use your thumbs to make a rotating movement on each side of the spine to ease muscle tension (Fig. 21c). Then stroke gently up to the back of the neck several times, using each hand alternately.

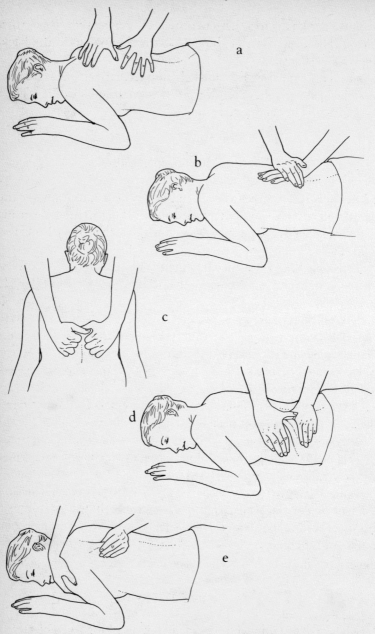

Fig. 21. Back massage sequence.

Press your hands together enclosing soft connective tissue, then release (Fig. 21d). Start at the buttocks and move up to the back. Repeat on other side.

Lift each shoulder slightly and lightly squeeze the tissue around the shoulder blades to relieve tension; press down firmly (Fig. 21e). Then massage with circular movements.

The Two-Minute Face Reviver

It takes only two minutes a day to massage your skin to stimulate the circulation and give yourself a healthy glow. Do this after cleansing your skin either in the morning or evening to make you look and feel great (Fig. 22).

First, apply a fluid moisturizer or light oil. Use both hands to sweep out to the sides and move up from the neck to your forehead (Fig. 24 on page 85).

If you are doing this massage in the morning, gently pinch your face from cheekbone to jaw line, then, using your index fingers, make circular movements on the sides of your nose and up over the eyebrows. Press for two seconds on the inner and outer corners of eyes and at the eyebrows.

To improve the blood supply to the skin's surface, tap your fingers over your face, from your neck up to under your eyes.

Next, stroke from your brows to the hairline, using both your index fingers. Stroke rapidly in the morning to wake you up; use slower movements at night to slow you down.

To finish off, place both hands together over your nose and mouth, then gently smooth over your face several times. In the morning, do this quickly to revive skin; slowly at night to soothe. You will soon notice the difference!

Other Massage Techniques

A daily work-out with 5 minutes of dry skin brushing will whisk away dead skin cells, help the lymph glands to flush out internal toxins, which are the cause of cellulite, and smooth rough, pimply skin. Using a good, firm natural bristle brush, firmly brush all over the body with upward strokes, starting at the soles of the feet. Do this before your daily bath or shower, and concentrate on the hips and thighs to disperse cellulite and improve skin texture (Fig. 23). (See also Appendix 2, pages 110–12.)

If you feel exhausted, try stimulating your adrenal glands by means of a pressure point on your palm. If you trace a straight line across the palm beginning at your thumb and drop another line from the join between your index and second fingers. The pressure point for your adrenal gland is where the two lines meet. Gently press on the area for 30 seconds with your index finger. Do the same for the other hand.

Improve your circulation and reduce cellulite by using a massage mitt in the bath or shower. Stroke in long, sweeping movements, working towards the heart.

Ease tension from face with a massage with a light facial oil (do not use an essential oil). Cleanse your face, then use your fingers to dot the oil over your face and neck. Starting at the neck, smooth upwards with the pads of your fingers, going up over the chin and using small circular movements around the nose. Carefully smooth around the eyes and towards the nose, finally stroke across forehead. Then stand on your head for a few seconds to improve your circulation. This will re-energize your whole body!

REFLEXOLOGY

Reflexologists believe that each part of the body has a corresponding area on the face, hands or feet. By massaging these points, the reflex zones, any tensions that may be blocking the internal flow of energy are released. Reflexology will also eliminate waste matter that may have accumulated in the body because of ill health or stress. It will eliminate stress, which is a major factor in as much as 75 per cent of

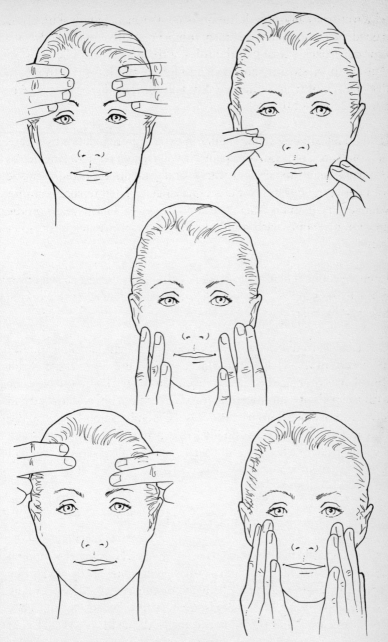

Fig. 22.   *Two minute face reviver.*

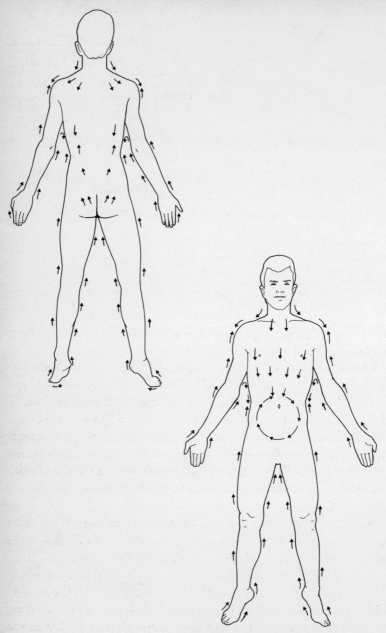

Fig. 23.   Dry skin brushing.

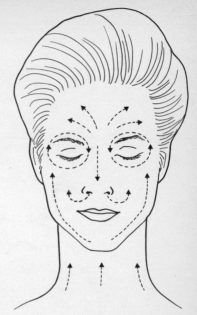

Fig. 24. Oiling the face and neck.

all illnesses. It also increases blood flow to the body's organs and improves general vitality and health.

Reflexology will also assist in ridding the body of toxins, the waste products from alcohol, red meat, caffeine, tannin (in tea) and cigarettes, which your body cannot get rid of itself. Instead of flushing them out of its system, your body stores them in deposits, which are dispersed only slowly and passed out of the body unnoticed. If more toxins than the body can cope with enter the system, the body has difficulty breaking them down, and the deposits can lead to health and beauty problems such as dull skin and hair and the build-up of deposits of cellulite.

As well as performing a daily foot massage (see page 87) to assist in breaking up these deposits, you should also try to eliminate the above toxin-causing products for at least two days once a month.

Reflexology pressure points are located in the face, hands and feet. Look at the diagrams on pages 86-9 and concentrate on the areas in which you have a problem. If, for example, you have a weak bladder, pay particular attention to this pressure point on the face, hands and feet. If you work on all three reflex zones for at least a total of 15

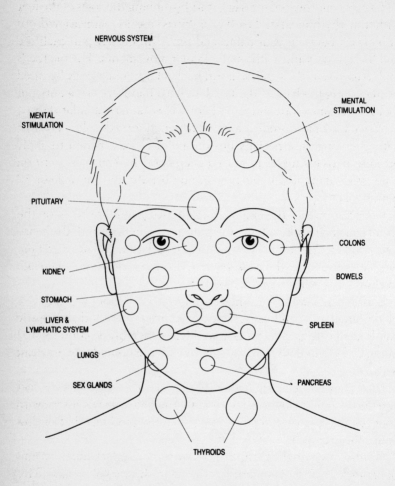

NERVOUS SYSTEM

MENTAL STIMULATION

MENTAL STIMULATION

PITUITARY

COLONS

KIDNEY

BOWELS

STOMACH

LIVER & LYMPHATIC SYSYEM

SPLEEN

LUNGS

SEX GLANDS

PANCREAS

THYROIDS

Fig. 25. Reflexology zones in the face.

minutes every day, you will notice an improvement in your general health within a week.

To carry out the foot massage, start by rubbing the soles of the feet with firm, rhythmical strokes. If your skin is very dry, warm a few drops of body oil between your palms and rub it in. Gently pull each toe and loosen the joints with small circular movements. The big toe is said to represent the head, so a stiff neck and shoulders may be eased by massaging the base of the toe. Use both hands to wring out your foot like a damp cloth and tap it lightly to stimulate circulation.

When you practise reflexology, try to penetrate as deeply as possible with your fingers, especially on sore points. Use a pencil to apply pressure if your fingers do not go deep enough. You must perform reflexology daily if you are to gain any benefit and for at least 10 minutes a day.

Use a hairbrush – the kind with cushioned points are best – on the top of feet and hands, in long sweeping movements towards the heart, for a total of 5 minutes. This improves circulation and assists reflexology massage to get the body's systems working effectively again and to eliminate toxins from the blood.

Elastic bands wound on the ends of fingers and toes will improve blood circulation and assist reflexology massage. Wind the elastic bands as tightly as you can bear and leave them in position for 1–2 minutes. Do this daily, making sure that all fingers and toes are dealt with.

If you have an electric body massager, use this on your face, feet and hands in place of, or in addition to, the reflexology massage with your fingers. Use on full power for your hands and feet, but on low power for your face.

While you are in the bath, scrub the soles of your feet and the palms of hands with a wet body brush lathered in shower gel or soap. This will stimulate circulation and keep the skin smooth for the maximum effectiveness of the reflexology massage.

Reflexology – A Word of Caution

Reflexology is a medical treatment and you should, therefore only go

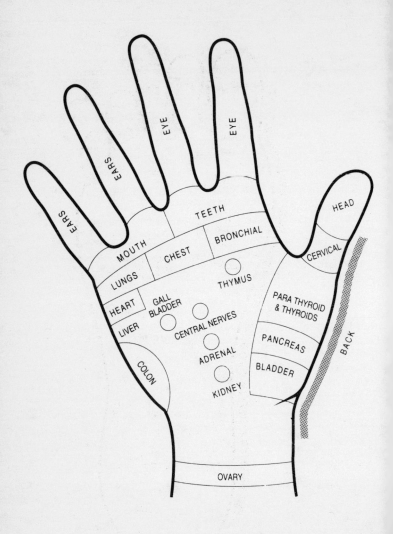

Fig. 26. *Reflexology zones in the hand.*

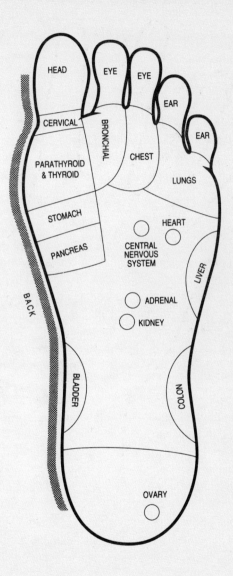

Fig. 27. Reflexology zones in the foot.

to a trained practitioner, preferably one recommended by the International Institute of Reflexology (for address see Useful Addresses on page 115).

Never perform reflexology on anyone who is diagnosed with thrombosis, as it can cause the clot to move. Epileptics should also avoid this therapy.

Reflexology picks up slight imbalances and can cause unnecessary alarm. For example, everyone will feel tenderness in kidney and adrenal areas, but this does not necessarily mean that they have kidney or adrenal trouble. For example, people who drink a lot of tea or coffee will appear to have kidney trouble, but the tenderness goes away soon after they give these up.

AROMATHERAPY

Aromatherapy involves massaging selected essential oils, diluted in a carrier oil (e.g. almond or wheatgerm), into the body, particularly the head, shoulders, spine and feet. As well as affecting the entire nervous system, aromatherapy has two other effects, one on your sense of smell, the other on the sense of touch.

Essential oils are sensuously soothing. Lavender and neroli are especially good for insomnia. Make sure you get your beauty sleep by massaging a few drops (diluted) on to your skin or put a few drops on a tissue and slip it under the pillow.

Do not be tempted to use oils indiscriminately just because they are natural and widely available. Some oils, such as sage and thyme, can be extremely toxic; too much marjoram can be narcotic; peppermint can cause dizziness; and eucalyptus may cause skin irritations. In fact sage, thyme, cinnamon bark and basil oils should not be sold to the public.

Essential oils last about a year, although they will last for twice as long if they are kept in the fridge. They should be well wrapped up to prevent their taking in other flavours. Most blended oils last for 3 months, but if wheatgerm oil was used as the carrier they will last for a year as wheatgerm is a natural preservative. Do not use an oil that is cloudy or smells weak, because it has gone off. Essential oils must always be kept in a dark place in a dark glass bottle with a stopper top. Do not keep oils in the bathroom, because they evaporate and go off in a steamy atmosphere.

The following herbal oils can be used by adding a few drops to steam and inhaling them through the nose for maximum efficiency. Tangerine is an anti-depressant; peppermint oil is good for colds; and eucalyptus oil clears up blocked noses, sinuses and sore throats.

The following oils can be used in steam, but not inhaled, or diluted in carrier oil and applied to the skin with your fingers:

Wheatgerm oil is good for dry skin;
Evening primrose oil has anti-wrinkle properties;
Almond oil is a good moisturizer;
Lavender oil added to the bath is relaxing and soothing;
Coconut oil can be massaged into the hair to cure dandruff and a scaly scalp (leave it on for an hour so that it can penetrate, then wash off thoroughly).

Blending Oils

There are no fixed rules about blending oils for aromatherapy. The oils can be used on their own, although aromatherapists believe that they work better if they are blended with other oils. You should never use any aromatherapy oil neat on your skin nor should you ever ingest an aromatherapy oil. They are very powerful, volatile substances and could be dangerous if used inappropriately (see pages 93-4). For more detailed and comprehensive information on aromatherapy I strongly recommend Christine Wildwood's book *Health Essentials: Aromatherapy* (which is published by Element Books).

To begin with, try blending oils of the same general kind – herbs (basil, clary-sage, lavender, marjoram and rosemary), citrus (bergamot, lemon and orange), flowers (rose, ylang-ylang and camomile) or spices (coriander and ginger). The easiest and most economical way to experiment is to put a few drops of essential oil on a roll of damp cotton wool. Then make up your favourite blend, keeping always to the same proportions.

Blending Treatment Oils

Problem	Essential oils	Application method
Aching muscles	Lavender, juniper	Baths, massage
Acne	Camomile, juniper	Facial oil, steam
Anxiety	Bergamot, camomile	Baths, massage
Arthritis	Camomile, cypress	Baths, massage
Burns and scalds	Lavender	Apply neat
Catarrh	Lavender, myrrh	Baths, steam
Cellulite	Juniper, cypress	Baths, massage
Colds, sinusitis	Juniper, eucalyptus	Baths, steam
Constipation	Rose, marjoram	Baths, massage
Dandruff	Camomile, juniper	Scalp massage
Depression	Bergamot, camomile	Baths, massage
Gingivitis	Tea tree, myrrh	Mouthwash
Headache	Camomile, lavender	Head/face massage
High blood pressure	Lavender	Baths, massage
Insect stings	Lavender, tea tree	Apply neat
Insomnia	Bergamot, camomile	Baths, massage
Menopause	Cypress, geranium	Baths, massage
Pre-menstrual syndrome/period pains	Geranium, juniper	Massage, baths

Blending oils will not only improve their fragrance but will also enhance their holistic effect. For example, if you are suffering from depression, with its associated side-effects of insomnia, anxiety and tense muscles, you will blend an anti-depressant such as lavender with a muscle relaxant such as pine-needle and a touch of ylang-ylang to uplift your spirits.

The chart on this page suggests which oils can be blended to help treat a variety of minor ailments. Please refer to the section Aromatherapy – A Word of Caution at the bottom of page 93 before blending oils.

Massage Tips

Aromatherapy massage can be done by a partner or friend, or you can do the head and feet massage yourself.

Use a bought massage oil or your favourite aromatherapy oil, making sure that you have studied the list of oils in the Aromatherapy Oils to be used with Caution (see page 94) before you start.

If you have a back problem, be careful – a massage could make it worse.

Do not massage over varicose veins or bruises.

Massage can help to spread infection and irritate inflamed areas.

Avoid therapists offering 'slimming' massages; massage alone cannot help you lose weight. It is best to go to your doctor for advice before embarking on a slimming programme.

Aromatherapy – A Word of Caution

Aromatherapy is the most popular of all the complementary therapies, because the combined effects of aromatic scents and relaxing massage give a very pleasant sensation.

However, before you go to a professional aromatherapist or try self-massage, you should be aware of the potential dangers and limitations of the therapy. Remember that anyone can set up as an aromatherapist; you should go to an aromatherapist recommended by the International Federation of Aromatherapists (the address of which is given under Useful Addresses, see page 115).

Aromatherapists should never recommend that oils be taken internally. Two deaths from poisoning with essential oils have been reported in the medical press. Oils can build up toxic levels in the body over a period of time, and because essential oils penetrate the skin, they can easily get into the bloodstream and have a profound effect on the kidneys. Do not use them if you are undergoing chemotherapy or homoeopathy, as they will cancel out the effects of those treatments. See the chart (page 94) to see which oils should be avoided.

Aromatherapy can help cellulite (see page 112), but the treatment must be supported by the right diet and exercise. Lymphatic drainage massage is used, which helps to eliminate toxic materials from the body, and this should be carried out only by qualified aromatherapists.

Aromatherapy Oils to be Used with Caution

Oil	Can cause
Basil, lemon, lemongrass	Skin irritation
Bergamot, cumin, lemon	Skin sensitivity to ultraviolet light
Black pepper, cardamon	Urinary/digestive problems
Cinnamon, fennel, thyme	Irritation/sensitive skin
Fennel, sage	Epileptic fits
Sage	Miscarriage
Sage, thyme	High blood pressure

6

Healthy Diet, Healthy Skin

A good diet is essential for a healthy skin. Your diet should contain a good mix of vegetables, pulses and fruit. Try to eat food that is fresh and is prepared immediately before it is eaten. Remember that vegetables are at their most nutritious if they are eaten raw.

Drinking at least six glasses of fresh water a day will help to flush waste and impurities from your body and keep skin clear. Protein is essential for building up strong and healthy connective tissue, which is vital for keeping skin healthy. Vitamins C, A and D, which are present in fresh vegetables and fruit, are essential for the structure of the skin. Other important nutrients, such as calcium (which is good for teeth) and iron (which is essential for a healthy blood supply to the skin), are found in meat, dairy products and fresh vegetables; they may not be present in over-processed convenience and frozen foods.

When you are planning individual recipes, think about your overall dietary needs for the week ahead. If you consider your evening meal is your main meal of the day, each week can contain the following evening meals: one poultry dish, two meat dishes, one fish dish, two vegetable dishes and one recipe based on pulses. A vegetarian diet is very healthy and vegetarians or vegans can stick to the same principles by using substitutes for animal protein such as soya, tofu, pulses and cheeses. These dishes should be served with fresh salads as starters and fresh fruit for desert. Fruit juice cocktails or mineral water are the healthy alternatives to alcohol with your meal.

Applying these principles, a typical weekly menu is on page 96. Leave your favourite recipes for the weekend, when you will have more time to enjoy them. Try to alternate between the light dishes, such as vegetables, pulses and fish, with the heavier dishes of poultry and meat.

Typical Weekly Menu

Monday: A pulse recipe
Tuesday: Meat dish
Wednesday: Pizza
Thursday: Chicken dish
Friday: Fish dish
Saturday: Vegetable dish
Sunday: Meat dish with rice

The ways in which you cook and garnish the dishes can be varied to suit your individual taste, but by having poultry, fish, meat, vegetables and pulses every week, you will have variety and balance, both essential for a healthy diet.

If you have a cooked evening meal, your lunch should be light – sandwiches, perhaps, with salad, meat, poultry or fish fillings. Do not make the mistake of skipping breakfast; a quick cooked recipe should be a good start to the day. There are plenty of excellent 'healthy food' cookbooks on the market which should give you plenty of inspiration!

Remember to drink at least six glasses of water, preferably mineral water, every day. Avoid alcoholic drinks altogether and cut down your consumption of tea and coffee. The best drinks by far are natural, unsweetened fruit juices.

A HEALTHY DIET

Keeping up with a hectic lifestyle demands a healthy diet. In today's fast paced world it is essential to eat nourishing simple food to maintain energy levels.

A healthy diet should include all the necessary requirements of protein, carbohydrate and a small amount of fat, as well as vitamins and minerals. Refined and overprocessed foods deplete the body of nutrients and destroy vitamins, such as vitamin D. In addition, they sometimes contain poisonous additives.

The easiest way to eat a healthy diet is to eat food in its natural state. For example, the healthiest way to eat fruit is when it is raw; the processes of tinning or preserving fruit deplete essential nutrients. Similarly, foods such as meat and vegetables should be purchased fresh. Eating and cooking fresh food, rather than overprocessed foods, will help you to build up your body's defences and reduce the incidence of allergies.

Eating fresh foods is not only better for you from the point of view of the value of the food itself, but it will also help eliminate the huge amounts of sugar, salt and other extraneous ingredients that manufacturers add to processed foods, not to mention the unnecessary additives such as colourings, flavourings and preservatives.

A Fat-Free Diet?

You will reduce the risk of becoming overweight by significantly reducing your fat intake. By preparing food yourself, you will also eliminate the unnecessary fat content of processed and refined foods, which not only contain high levels of hidden fat but also high levels of salt and sugar.

Adopt the following tips to promote a healthier you:

- Trim off all white fat from chicken, beef and lamb with a sharp knife. Purchase lean meat; although it may be more expensive, cheaper meat will contain more fat. To be completely sure of using lean mince, buy beef or lamb and trim off the fat before placing it in the mincer or food processor.

- Try to use the grill or cook in a microwave to reduce fat. The fat converts into a liquid, which can be poured away. If you do fry, use low-fat, low-cholesterol oil. Always drain food on a kitchen towel before serving to mop up any excess oil.

- Cook by steaming to avoid additional fat and to help retain nutrients and vitamins.

- Use low-fat ingredients in your cooking, such as low-fat butter blends or substitutes.

7

Making The Most of Your Make-up

The following tips and advice are based on my training as a make-up artist. I am always surprised at how inflexible people are when it comes to their make-up routines. They are only rarely willing to try new products, colours or textures but cling to their old style of make-up. The key to good make-up is experimentation, and the following information should help you rethink your make-up bag, routine and products.

Try to put on make-up only when it is absolutely necessary. Whenever you can, give your skin a break to allow it to breathe! Remember that make-up is made up of complex chemicals, perfumes and sometimes animal proteins and the by-products of industrial processes, such as petroleum refinement. Ask yourself if you really need to put it on when you are going out for a quick walk.

If you are a vegan or vegetarian – or if you are merely concerned about the contents of many beauty preparations – you may choose not to use beauty products or cosmetics of the mainstream ranges and to use instead ranges that state that they are suitable for vegetarians. Even with the specialist ranges, you cannot be 100 per cent sure of their contents, so you may wish to write to the different cosmetic companies to ask which of their products do not contain animal tissue. For example, many lipsticks contain slaughterhouse by-products such as pig fat, while many anti-wrinkle creams contain animal proteins. Even the so-called 'natural' products can contain lanolin, which is derived from sheep's wool.

In Britain the contents of cosmetics do not have to be shown, although legislation will be introduced for compulsory labelling by the mid-1990s. In the United States, however, all the contents of cosmetics have, by law, to be shown. Lipsticks may contain the following ingredients: castor oil, candelilla wax, beeswax, lanolin, animal protein, lecithin, fragrance and colours such as iron oxides. Phew, all that in one lipstick! Vegetarians should note the inclusion of animal protein and ask whether using it conflicts with their values.

Do you need to put on all these ingredients? And how often do you need to wear them? Try to avoid wearing make-up unless it is absolutely necessary. If you work full-time, of course, make-up will certainly give your ego a boost, but when you are at home, try to go without it. When you do wear make-up, try to limit the range and number of products that you use. Select products that contain natural ingredients or products designed for sensitive skins, which do not contain perfume or irritants.

When you consider the number of complex chemicals that go into cosmetics, it is not surprising that they can cause allergic reactions. Some products are so harsh that they harm the acid mantle, the protective layer of the skin that keeps it healthy and soft, and so make the skin more sensitive and blemish prone. If you must use make-up products in your daily routine, try to use them sparsely, and apply with a gentle touch to the skin.

PERFECT MAKE-UP

Well applied make-up is perfectly blended and symmetrical, has no hard edges or harsh lines, and looks as natural as possible. The key to applying make-up successfully is experimentation. It is only by experimenting with different looks, colours and products, that you will find the look that bests suits you and with which you are most confident. The reason why models look so great is that they have experienced hundreds of different looks and, after all that experimentation, have found a look that matches their personality and features.

Think about the occasions on which you have been complimented on your make-up. Write down the exact compliment, if you can remember it. What colours were they, shiny or matte? What form of application did you use? Try to build up an idea of the look that others liked on you. Did you yourself feel more confident with these looks?

Each individual feels comfortable with particular colours. This is why when you have a professional make-over, you may not be entirely happy with the result. The make-up artist does not know which colours suit you, both physically and chemically. Colours emit different energy levels that can be synchronized with certain individuals, not just to match their eye, hair and skin colour. There are, for example, cold and warm colours. Red is a hot colour that emits high energy levels; blue and grey are cool colours, which are calming and relaxing.

Buying Cosmetics

Try to limit the number of 'corrective' products that you buy. For example, if you find yourself using a concealer to cover problem skin, it would be better to correct the skin by means of facials or special treatments, such as the specific skin treatments described in Chapter 2. There is nothing more false than having a thick mask on your face.

Some concealers and foundation creams can actually accentuate lines and wrinkles, while grease-based preparations can aggravate oiliness, so making the skin worse. If you have dark shadows under the eyes, get some sleep! If they become permanent, they could indicate a nutritional deficiency or ill health. See your doctor, rather than continually relying on concealer to disguise the symptom.

The new all-in-one foundation/powders can reduce the need for foundation and powder make-up base. They are excellent for young skins and good complexions; however, they can make mature faces look older and problem skins worse. Some can look 'cakey'; others give light coverage. If you are unsure whether these products are for you, try the cheapest brand or look out for small samples or trial sizes. Some of the manufacturers of more expensive cosmetics include small sizes of their foundation/powder compacts in promotional offers, so look out for these.

The cosmetic and perfumery counters of most large department stores often have demonstration sizes, so have a good try and do not be intimidated by the beauty consultant. Tell her what you need and your specific problems, and she will generally be able to offer good advice.

Applying Make-Up

Avoid ending up with a chalky face by shaking a little loose powder into the palm of your hand and using a soft powder puff or a cotton wool ball to pat and roll the powder gently on to your skin. When you have covered your entire face, take a large brush and dust off the excess, paying particular attention to the crevices around your nose, eyes and chin.

For a perfect, flawless finish, always apply foundation with a soft, synthetic sponge. Smoothing foundation with your fingers can transfer bacteria to your skin and encourage infection. Natural sponges also tend to harbour bacteria as they are difficult to wash. Always wash your make-up sponge after each use with warm, soapy water.

If you are fed up with feeling that your make-up never looks quite right, try a free make-over at a professional make-up school, where make-up artists train. You will receive good advice and can experiment with lots of new looks and products.

MAKING THE PERFECT SHADE FROM YOUR EXISTING FOUNDATION

Foundations come in so many different textures and combinations that it is very easy to make mistakes. The foundation you use should blend in with your natural colouring so that it looks as though you are not wearing any! Your colouring will not exactly match the colour of the foundation, so it is sensible to spend some time creating your own foundation to match your skin.

The key to getting the exact colour combination for your skin, is experimentation. For your initial experiments you may prefer to use the cheaper products to limit the cost of your mistakes. Some cosmetic counters may give out free samples, especially of new lines, or you may want to try the teenage end of the market, where products are budget priced.

You will need to use at least three foundations to create your individual colour. If you are pale, stick to two or three of the palest colours in the range; if you are dark, pick foundations from the darker end of the range, adding one pale shade to lighten the mix if it gets too dark. If your colouring is medium, pick one pale, one medium and one dark colour, all from the same range.

You can, of course, try blending the foundations that are already in your make-up bag, but you will probably find that they do not blend easily with each other. For example, if one is dewy moisturizing foundation and one is a matte, oil-free foundation, each will offset the effect of the other. So, if possible, stick to colours from the same range. Liquid foundations are best for blending, as well as being ideal for oily and black skins, some being oil-absorbent.

Lay out the foundations on a clear table. Have ready a few clean, flat saucers for blending, together with a few teaspoons. You will also need a notebook and pen with which to note down the different combinations you are blending. Have a clear bottle ready to store your exact shade of foundation when you have finished experimenting.

Start mixing different combinations of the foundations, making a note of each one. Try to be precise – that is, if you have used one spoon of shade A to two spoons of shade B, note this down exactly. When you have three or four mixes, put them on your cheek/jawline area in thick strips with a lip brush in good light. Critically assess which foundation is best.

If the foundations do not match your skin, try blending again until you reach the perfect combination. Make a note of the exact combination and blend them in exactly the same proportions to make a full size bottle. There you have it, the perfect foundation for your skin colouring!

CREATING NEW COLOURS FROM YOUR EXISTING LIPSTICKS

If you are bored with your existing lipsticks or cannot afford to buy new shades, fear not. You can use your existing lipsticks to create literally hundreds of combinations of new and existing colours. All you need is the back of your hand (for blending), a lip brush and your existing lipsticks. It is best to have a varied colour spectrum, including reds, pinks, oranges, browns, gold, violets and blue-reds.

If you do not have some of the lipsticks from the basic ranges, you may want to ask friends if they have some spare lipsticks that they are not using. The wider the initial range of colours you use, the more shades you will be able to create. Simply blend the colours on the back of your hand with a lip brush, taking some lipstick from each of your chosen shades, and apply the 'new' shade directly to your lips. You may want to experiment with three or four combinations before you decide on one to try on your lips.

You can also co-ordinate lipsticks with your clothes; for example, if a blouse is salmon pink, blend brown with a pink lipstick. If a dress has a special shade of red in it, you can highlight it by creating the exact shade of red lipstick!

TAILORING MAINSTREAM MAKE-UP TO SUIT BLACK WOMEN

As black skins tend to vary in colour, finding an exact shade to match your complexion colour can be a problem. Cosmetics specially made for 'black' women are often unsatisfactory, as their quality and performance are still poor. In addition, because of the smaller volumes sold, their prices are also far from competitive.

One solution is to look for specific colours in the mainstream range of the major make-up houses. These companies now produce foundations, powders and bronzing powders intended to give a fake 'sun-tanned look', which can work very well with darker skins. Most ranges will incorporate three or four shades, which vary according to the strength of the 'tan', so if you are very dark skinned, you may wish to try the deepest fake tan product. The fairer your skin is, the more you can get away with using most of the colours in mass-market ranges catering for Europeans.

Remember that your eyeshadow, lipstick and blusher should just be a tone darker than your skin tone to achieve a natural finish. This means that if you have a very dark skin, you should use deep browns, reds and possibly peach colours to achieve a natural look.

A good make-up base begins with a good foundation that *exactly* matches your individual skin colour. Never try to use a foundation that is a shade lighter than your natural colour; it will look mask-like and unnatural. Unless you are very fair, you should at all cost avoid the ivories and pale beiges that are intended for European women. Here is the easiest way to tailor-make foundation and powder from the main ranges to suit your exact colour:

- Sit in a brightly coloured room in front of a very large mirror. Look at your skin colour critically. What is the overall tone? Is there any underlying colour such as red?

- For your experiments you will need three or four foundations and/or powders from the cheapest mainstream range, ranging from the lightest to the darkest, including 'sun' ranges. Now, make at least ten different combinations of the colours.

- Brush the mixed foundations in patches on to the cheek and jaw area. Look in good light to decide which combination closely matches your own.

Blend a larger quantity of the combination that best suits you and put this foundation in a clean jar or bottle. You can now use this foundation whenever you wish without having to worry about the 'natural' look.

Once you have gained the confidence to make your own individual foundation with cheap products, you can progress to the more expensive ranges, as they will give better coverage. You can apply the same concept to powder, which again should match your skin tone if it is not to look very chalky, and to eye shadows, blushers and, of course, lipsticks. Remember that two or three lipsticks can combine together to produce a shade that will match your skin tone perfectly.

By mixing together different products, you can create a 'natural' look that may not have been possible by simply purchasing 'black' make-up. Have fun experimenting!

MATCHING MAKE-UP COLOURS WITH YOUR SKIN TONE

Have you ever looked at the glossy advertisements and features pages of magazines and copied the make-up look exactly only to find out that it did not suit you? The make-up may have looked wonderful with the model's skin, hair, eye colour and features, but it will not necessarily have suited your individual colouring.

Only certain colours will suit a particular combination of colouring of skin, hair and eyes. To help you choose the colours that suit you, look at the different groups listed below and decide to which of them you belong. The groups are not rigid, and there is room for overlap between them. Then try the colours on your face and make a note of the colour group that suits you best. Ask a close friend for an opinion – but make sure he or she is honest!

- *Group 1: Light beige, dark 'black' or olive skin, grey/green/brown eyes, dark hair* – Make-up of deep blue-pinks and blue-reds, with cool eyeshadows in greys, blues and purples.

- *Group 2: Pink-beige skin, light 'black', neutral beige 'Asian' skin, grey/blue eyes, brown hair* – Make-up in soft, gentle pinks or mauves with eyeshadows in sea blue and sea green.

- *Group 3: Ivory skin (rarely black or Asian skin), green eyes, red hair* – Make-up in coppery reds and brown-peach, and eyeshadows in green, brown and deep earthy green.

- *Group 4: Ivory, golden 'black', very light Asian skin, blue eyes, blonde hair* – Make-up in warm colours such coral pinks, peaches, bright red, and eyeshadows in yellow, pink, blue, and green.

106

BEAUTY PROBLEMS THAT MAKE-UP CANNOT DISGUISE

There are some beauty problems that even perfect make-up, applied by the best make-up artists, cannot disguise. Your face is a good indicator of your state of health and well-being so you cannot be beautiful if you are not healthy. There are nerve endings below the skin of your face, so if you are feeling below par it is not surprising that this shows up in your face.

Stress and pollution, which may have had adverse effects on your health, will leave their marks on your face for the whole world to see. No matter how clever you are with make-up, you cannot disguise these lines and wrinkles nor the underlying ill health. You have only to step into a hospital to look at the faces of people who have been seriously ill to realize that neither the best make-up products nor the finest techniques could make them look the picture of health, although make-up could make them look better and improve their confidence.

Stress and ill health will affect your whole body and therefore your face, but a specific illness will manifest itself on the specific nerve endings in the skin of the face. Bad skin can almost always be equated with bad health. Spot-prone and problem skin can often be linked to stress as well as to poor digestive and waste disposal systems, such as the stomach and kidneys. A pasty complexion may signify problems with the bowels. In such cases, rather than trying to disguise these problems, it is much better to seek advice from your doctor to deal with the underlying cause.

Similarly, persistent dark circles under your eyes do not always indicate a lack of sleep. They can be the result of poor diet or nutrient deficiency or they may simply be hereditary. It is much better to check with your doctor before piling on the concealer.

Make-up cannot disguise a poor self-image, which is built up over the years, particularly in childhood, and is deeply ingrained in the mind. By carrying out the treatments in this book, you will go a step towards improving your self-image. The problem with incorrectly applied make-up, however, is that it can reinforce your self-image. If you have small eyes, you will naturally go overboard with eye make-up. Unfortunately, you will actually bring attention to your small eyes rather than make them look larger. Bold eyeliner, incorrectly applied, will make eyes look smaller. The trick is to highlight each of your features evenly by accentuating the good – full lips, for example – and hiding the bad – small eyes, for example.

Make-up cannot disguise prominent features. There is a technique of using light and dark shades of foundation to 'correct' features, with light shades highlighting 'good' areas and dark shades hiding the 'bad'. In principle, the theory is correct, but in practice, it is easy to make mistakes and to end up looking artificial. You may even end up highlighting the very feature you wanted to conceal. It is better to forget such 'corrective' techniques, and just concentrate on your best features – for example, if you have lovely eyes, spend extra time making the most of them.

Some people are unfortunate enough to have permanent birth-marks or port wine stains on visible parts of their face or body. Applying make-up to conceal them requires special training, and rather than trying to patch up the area yourself you should ask your general practitioner to refer you to a specialist who will be able to suggest the appropriate products to use and offer expert advice.

The use of make-up in certain circumstances is, as we have seen, limited but I hope that this will not deter you from having fun experimenting with make-up. Nevertheless, always remember that if you have problems that are more than superficial – that are not just skin deep – you should find the underlying reasons, rather than continuing the uphill struggle of achieving perfection with make-up.

Appendix 1: Natural Depilation

In the Middle East it is customary for all the bride's body hair to be removed before the marriage ceremony. This is done using only natural products such as water, sugar, lemon juice and honey.

One method that is widely used is sugaring, which involves the use of nothing more than water and sugar, heated gently, in different proportions, depending on the preference of the user. Sugaring can be tricky to perfect, but the time spent practising will eventually save time and money and will give smooth, stubble-free skin, which will remain hair-free for up to 8 weeks.

Try the 1:1 technique to start off with; mix 1 tablespoon (20 ml) of water with 1 tablespoon (20 ml) of granulated sugar in a metal pan, over gentle heat. When the sugar has dissolved and the liquid is the consistency of honey, allow it to cool slightly and, when it reaches body temperature, apply it with a wooden spoon or spatula. Press the mixture on to your skin with your hands or use a strip of cotton. Allow it to set then pull it off with your hands or lift off the cotton, remembering to pull against the direction in which the hair grows. Rinse your skin with cold water.

You can vary the proportions of sugar to water depending on how thick you like the mixture and the consistency you find easiest to work with. Once you are familiar with the technique, you can make larger amounts in the same proportions of sugar to water. You may find it messy at first, but after practice, it will be fuss and mess free! You will notice that the method leaves a lovely sheen on the skin.

Alternatively, you may want to try warming the juice of a small lemon or half a large lemon with 10 tablespoons (200 ml) of granulated sugar. Warm the mixture until the sugar dissolves and continue as before. You may find this technique easier to do.

Another recipe, which is good for dry skins is to use 1 tablespoon (20 ml) of water, 1 tablespoon (20 ml) of sugar, 1 dessertspoon (10 ml) of real lemon juice and 1 teaspoon (5 ml) of honey. Warm the mixture until sugar dissolves and continue as above. The moisturizing properties in the honey soften dry skin.

If you shave your legs, you will need to do it every three or four days, and you will have stubble. The above methods leave no stubble. Whichever method of depilation you use, you will find that it helps to exfoliate too, leaving your skin fresher as well as hair free.

The best and easiest way to remove hair on your legs is by investing in a long-lasting electrical coil, which acts like a tweezer and removes hair from the root. There is no stubble and the effects last for up to six weeks. Some women find the method painful at first, but they quickly get accustomed to it. If you find the process difficult, minimize the pain by wiping the area with a flannel soaked in ice-cold water (to de-sensitize it) and holding the skin taut.

Appendix 2: Treatments for Cellulite

You do not need expensive treatments, gels or equipment to get rid of cellulite; you can do it for free by following the simple treatments below. Be persistent, carry out the routines daily and be patient: the results will soon become evident.

It may help you to monitor your measurements, so before you begin measure your waist, hips, thighs and arms, holding the tape measure around the fullest part (you may need the help of your partner or a friend). Write the measurements down in your diary together with the date. When you are carrying out the treatments daily, you should make a note of your measurements weekly, and you should see them gradually decrease. Even if there is no decrease, you will still note the improvement in the texture and firmness of the skin.

Keep a watch on your diet, too, because you do not want to consume unnecessary fat. You may also want to keep a check of your overall weight when you are taking your weekly measurements. Flushing out toxins from your body, should also result in a decrease in weight. Increasing the exercise you take, such as jogging, cycling or swimming, should also assist in dislodging stubborn cellulite.

Daily dry skin brushing before your bath or shower will increase your blood circulation and help lymphatic drainage, so getting rid of accumulated toxins, which are the cause of hard cellulite areas. Choose a good firm brush and beginning at the thighs, brush in long,

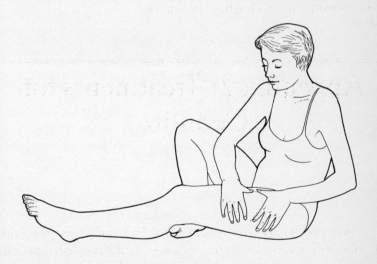

Fig. 28.   Self-massage for cellulite.

sweeping movements towards the heart. On areas of stubborn cellulite use circular movements and increased pressure.

The buttocks are an area in which the 'orange peel' skin typical of cellulite can accumulate. Pay particular attention to this area by vigorous scrubbing with your brush, continuing with upward sweeping movements. If you have cellulite around your abdomen, circle in vigorous movements, as well as towards your heart. To treat cellulite on your arms, raise arms straight up in the air and, with long, sweeping movements, brush downwards towards the heart, concentrating on specific areas of cellulite.

After doing this routine for 5–10 minutes daily, shower and bath as usual. You will note that your skin will be extra soft, because brushing has the added advantage of dislodging dead skin cells as well as bringing the blood supply to the surface of the skin, ensuring good skin condition. Combine the brushing routine with the following massage technique for maximum effect.

Massage Techniques

Using your fingers, massage areas of cellulite as if you were kneading dough. Cellulite will feel hard, but try to press your fingers as deeply as possible into the skin. Press for 10 seconds, then relax for 5 seconds.

You should endeavour to massage stubborn cellulite areas daily for at least 10 minutes. The areas should feel less hard with treatment and there should be fewer lumps. If you have an electric massage machine, use it daily to reduce cellulite build-up. Vibratory massage machines will relax and contract your muscles, assisting in reducing the accumulation of toxins and, therefore, cellulite.

Massaging your foot, hands and face (see the Reflexology section, pages 82–90) will help to make sure that the whole waste elimination system of the body (blood, kidneys, liver and lymph nodes) is working well to flush away harmful toxins from food, pollution and the body's internal processes.

Appendix 3: Achieving a Better Self-Image

Your self-image will have been developed during your childhood, and it stays with you throughout adulthood. If you have a poor self-image, you can improve it trying the effective treatments of relaxation, meditation and visualization.

RELAXATION

A poor self-image will reveal itself in a tense, tight body and a slumped, humped posture, which are the body language signals for low self-worth. Try relaxation techniques to get rid of this low self-esteem.

Close the curtains, unplug the telephone, lie down flat on the floor or on a bed in a darkened room, and do not answer the doorbell. Shut off all noise completely. Now gently breathe in, expanding your chest as far as it will go. Hold for a few seconds and gently breathe all of this out. Continue breathing in and out in this way for at least 10 minutes. You will feel instantly relaxed and on a 'high'.

MEDITATION

Meditation is an extension of the above relaxation technique. You can either lie down or sit with crossed legs. Start the gradual controlled breathing, and with each breath hum a short word; in meditation this is usually 'OM'. Continue for up to 30 minutes, and you will go into a trance-like state. The purpose of meditation is to rid the mind of the endless, and usually useless, chatter that goes on inside it, including negative thoughts about oneself. By focusing on repeating one word, you give the mind a well-earned break, and are re-energized and have a positive outlook.

VISUALIZATION

A powerful technique, visualization uses the power of the mind to create a positive self-image. Try to achieve a relaxed state, as in relaxation or meditation, then picture your ideal self in your mind. Make the picture very vivid. Now visualize your self-image. Use the powers of your mind to merge the two pictures together, and you will note that there is not much difference. Use this technique to overcome years of negative conditioning and to make your self-image in line with your ideal self.

Further Reading

Barlow, W., *The Alexander Principle*, Gollancz, 1990.
Brennan, R., *Health Essentials: The Alexander Technique*, Element Books, 1991.
Corvo, J., *Zone Therapy*, Century, 1990.
Cox and Dainton, *Making the Most of Yourself*, Sheldon, 1985.
Davies, P., *Your Total Image*, Piatkus, 1990.
Fraser, E., *Facial Workout*, Viking, 1990.
Guyton, A., *Woman's Book of Natural Beauty*, Thorsons, 1984.
Jackson, C., *Colour Me Beautiful, Make-up Book*, Piatkus, 1988.
Knox, N., *Beautiful Body, Beautiful Skin*, Piatkus, 1990.
Wildwood, C., *Health Essentials: Aromatherapy*; Element Books, 1991.
Wolf, N., *The Beauty Myth*, Vintage, 1990.

Useful Addresses

Complementary Medicine

For further information on complementary medicine contact:

The Institute For Complementary Medicine
PO Box 194
London SE16 1QZ

Reflexology

For an information leaflet on reflexology, a list of registered practitioners and a book list (£1) send a stamped addressed envelope to:

The International Institute of Reflexology
28 Hollyfield Avenue
London N11 3BY

For courses on reflexology contact:
The Bayly School of Reflexology
Monks Orchard
Whitbourne
Worcester WR6 5RB

For aromatherapy massage contact:
The Synergy Centre
1 Cadogan Gardens
London SW3

Aromatherapy

For a list of qualified practitioners in your area, send a stamped addressed envelope to:
International Federation of Aromatherapists
4 East Mearn Road
London SE21 8HA

International Federation of Aromatherapists
c/o Allison Russell
35 Bydown Street
Neutral Bay
New South Wales 2089
Australia

American Aromatherapy Association
PO Box 3609
Culver City
California 90231
USA

For information on aromatherapy contact the Tisserand Institute, the leading organization for research and education in the art of aromatherapy which runs courses and mail order services:
The Tisserand Institute
65 Church Road
Hove
Sussex PN3 2BD
Telephone 01273-206640

Massage

For massage courses contact:
The Northern Institute of Massage
100 Waterloo Road
Blackpool
Lancs FY4 1AW

Eczema

If you suffer from eczema contact:
The National Eczema Society
Tavistock House East
Tavistock Square
London WC1

Index